Cochlear Implants
for Young Children

This page is dedicated to our secretary, Liz Swainson, who patiently typed the manuscript. Our thanks are due to her for her patience.

Cochlear Implants for Young Children

The Nottingham Approach to Assessment and Rehabilitation

Edited by

Barry McCormick, PhD,

Sue Archbold, MPhil and Sarah Sheppard, MSc

Paediatric Cochlear Implant Programme, Nottingham

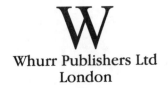

Whurr Publishers Ltd
London

© 1994 Whurr Publishers Ltd
First published 1994 by
Whurr Publishers Ltd
19b Compton Terrace, London N1 2UN, England

British Library Cataloguing in Publication Data
A catalogue record for this book is available from the
British Library.

ISBN 1-897635-80-X

Photoset by Stephen Cary
Printed and bound in the UK by Athenaeum Press Ltd,
Newcastle upon Tyne

Preface

The practice of paediatric cochlear implantation has grown at an exceptional pace over the 5 years before the publication of the book. This rapid development has placed demands on the teams to divide their time between the running of their programmes and the dissemination of information to professional colleagues and parents.

This book has been written to help satisfy the quest for knowledge about implantation in young children and to provide specific details about specialist techniques. It is hoped that the text will provide guidance and encouragement to other teams who may be considering the implantation of very young children. It should also be of value to students, professionals and parents who wish to acquaint themselves with knowledge about the issues and complexities in this rapidly expanding field.

Barry McCormick (Senior Editor)
December 1993

Contents

Contributors

Sue Archbold, MPhil, Paediatric Cochear Implant Programme, Nottingham, UK

Dee Dyar, LCSLT, Speech and Language Therapy Service, Nottingham, UK

Kevin P. Gibbin, FRCS, Department of Otolaryngology, Queen's Medical Centre, Nottingham, UK

Hazel Lloyd, BEd, Paediatric Cochlear Implant Programme, Nottingham, UK

Barry McCormick, PhD, Paediatric Cochlear Implant Programme, Nottingham, UK

Steve M. Mason, PhD, Medical Physics Department, Queen's Medical Centre, Nottingham, UK

Gerard M. O'Donoghue, FRCS, Department of Otolaryngology, Queens Medical Centre, Nottingham, UK

Mary Joe Osberger, PhD, Indiana University, Indiana, USA

Sarah Sheppard, MSc, Paediatric Cochlear Implant Programme, Nottingham, UK

Margaret Tait, PhD, Paediatric Cochlear Implant Programme, Nottingham, UK

Chapter 1
Introduction and overview

MARY JOE OSBERGER

In 1980, the first child was implanted with a single-channel cochlear prosthesis by William F. House, MD at the House Ear Institute in Los Angeles, California. Few people realised that this marked the beginning of a technological break-through in the management of profound hearing loss in children. Today, nearly 15 years after the first child was implanted, it has been established that cochlear prostheses provide considerable benefit to the development of speech perception and production skills in children with profound hearing impairments. Even though researchers strive to develop more effective implant processing schemes, the performance of children with the current technology has surpassed the expectations of most professionals and parents. In fact, no other sensory aid has had such a dramatic impact on improving the viability of oral communication for profoundly hearing-impaired children, not even acoustic amplification. Yet, even though the literature contains numerous research studies on children's performance with implants, the field is still in its infancy.

Paediatric work was preceded by successful use of the same devices by postlingually deafened adults. The adult research results revealed that single-channel implants provided improved sound detection and speechreading, but word recognition was limited. In contrast, adults' performance with more sophisticated devices (i.e. multichannel cochlear implants) revealed remarkable levels of word recognition. Many adults are able to understand speech without speechreading and some of them can communicate on the telephone. Even though adults demonstrated high levels of performance with multichannel cochlear implants, many professionals were apprehensive about the potential benefit of these devices for children. This concern arose because most children who are implant candidates acquired their deafness before speech and language were learned. Unlike postlingually deafened adults, who use the signal transmitted by an implant to compare with stored auditory representations of language, the prelingually deafened child must use the same signal to differentiate one auditory event from another, interpret meaning from such events, and organise and store this information for later access, retrieval and meaningful use. These are formidable tasks to accomplish with any auditory prosthesis given the exquisite temporal and frequency-resolving powers of the normal ear. On the other hand, young children might be successful at achieving high levels of performance with a cochlear prosthesis given the 'plasticity' of the central nervous system when many of them are implanted.

That children derived substantial benefit from electrical stimulation of the auditory system was demonstrated by the Food and Drug Administration's (FDA) approval of the Nucleus 22 channel cochlear implant for children on June 27 1990. This momentous decision helped to establish a permanent role for implants in children with profound hearing impairments. To date, the results have shown that roughly half of the children implanted with multichannel devices demonstrate some speech understanding without speechreading. Children who are unable to understand speech without speechreading can detect sound at lower (better) levels with an implant than they could with hearing aids, and they perceive the prosodic or rhythmic aspects of speech with an implant which were impossible to perceive with their hearing aids. Nearly every child demonstrates improved speechreading performance with an implant over what they had demonstrated with hearing aids. Children who are born deaf receive as much benefit from an implant as do children who acquired their deafness before the age of 3 years. There are, however, large individual differences among children in their performance with multichannel implants. One of the most important factors that explains differences between children is the length of time that they have used an implant. Research has shown that perception and production skills develop over a relatively long time course in prelingually deafened children. The performance of children has improved beyond 3 years of multichannel implant use, and the upper limit of performance with commercially available devices has not been established in children. As the performance of implanted children continues to improve over time, initial criteria used to determine implant candidacy have been challenged. Children who have some residual hearing in the profound range of impairment are now considered implant candidates and implants are now being recommended for very young, pre-verbal children which poses unique challenges in determining candidacy and device benefits.

In spite of the enormous enthusiasm about implants by most people, the use of these devices in children remains controversial for some. Those who are opposed to implants in children are members of the deaf community who do not view deafness as a handicap but as a cultural identity. According to this community, to restore hearing is to deny children their deaf heritage. Although the opinion of the deaf community is respected by professionals in the implant field, it is, nevertheless, the right of all parents to choose a course of action that they feel is in the best interest of their child. Given that most parents of deaf children hear normally and live in a hearing world, these parents have chosen an implant so that their child might have an opportunity to learn to talk and communicate with hearing as well as deaf people. Hearing parents' decisions to provide auditory input to their deaf child should also be respected.

To date, most of the paediatric implant literature consists of research findings on children's performance with the devices. There is an obvious lack of high-quality publications on the clinical and rehabilitative management of these children. Even though it is generally accepted that an implant team should be multidisciplinary in nature, relatively little is available that describes the components of such a team. This book was inspired by numerous requests made to the Nottingham Paediatric Cochlear Implant Group to provide an in-depth description of their team and the functions of each team member. In 1989, the first child was implanted in Nottingham and, since that time, a strong and cohesive multidisciplinary cochlear implant team has developed there. Within a relatively short period of time, a model implant programme has evolved in Nottingham which has gained international, as well as national, recognition. A unique aspect of the Nottingham approach is the extensive follow-up and training in each implanted child's home with their parents, and with the personnel in the child's school.

The book is intended for all those concerned with the assessment and habilitation of children with cochlear implants. The emphasis is on the management of young, pre-verbal children because they represent the largest, but most challenging, population of children who are implant candidates. A comprehensive overview of all aspects of the paediatric cochlear implant field is presented, beginning with a description (Chapter 2) of the basic design and components of cochlear implants and the processing strategies that are employed. Chapter 3 provides a conceptualisation of a paediatric cochlear implant team with the aims and objectives of the team developed taking the needs of the child and family into consideration. The next chapter, Chapter 4, presents an overview of audiological procedures to assess the hearing function and determine implant candidacy in young children – a challenging task for many audiologists who have limited experience with the paediatric population. The role of both behavioural and objective evaluation procedures is presented.

The medical and surgical aspects of implantation are presented in

Chapter 5 in terms of candidacy issues, surgical procedures, risks and complications. Ethical and consent issues, which are of particular importance in paediatric implant work, are also discussed in Chapter 5. As the implant fitting process is complex in young, pre-verbal children, information from objective tests such as the electric auditory brain-stem response (EABR) are invaluable in facilitating this process. The application of electrophysiological test results with the young paediatric population is discussed in Chapter 6. Completion of the psychophysical testing needed to set the implant requires special skills with the young, pre-verbal population. Device setting techniques which incorporate information obtained from stapedial reflex and EABR tests are described in Chapter 7.

In Chapter 8, habilitation techniques appropriate for young, pre-verbal children with profound hearing impairments are described. The authors provide a novel description of the stages of language development which occur in these young implanted children, with intervention techniques appropriate for each stage of development.

Chapters 9, 10 and 11 suggest methods of monitoring implant progress in terms of auditory, language and speech development respectively. These chapters provide details on the communication assessment methods used by this team, as well as valuable information on the type and rate of progress shown by young implanted children. The team employs databased procedures to monitor progress and develop intervention goals. Of particular interest is the structure of the programme in terms of the services provided in the child's home to the family and the personnel in the child's school. The approach taken by this team is to educate those people who spend the most time with the implanted child – the parents and teachers – so that they provide the continuous support services required by these children.

Finally, the last chapter describes family perspectives on implants. The parents of a number of implanted children provide valuable insight into the implant decision-making process, their reactions to deafness, and their struggles and triumphs in raising a child with a profound hearing impairment.

This book promises to provide professionals with a better understanding of the clinical aspects of the field of paediatric implantation which will help us provide a better service to the children and their families.

Chapter 2
Cochlear implant systems

SARAH SHEPPARD

Hearing impairment, and the consequent handicap and disability resulting from it, can be relieved in a variety of ways depending on the type, nature and degree of the hearing loss. The ear comprises the outer, middle and inner ear or cochlea (Figure 2.1). Dysfunction of the middle ear results in conductive hearing loss which is often temporary or treatable, but sensory hearing loss is caused by damage or malformation of the cochlea or the delicate structures within the cochlea; this is

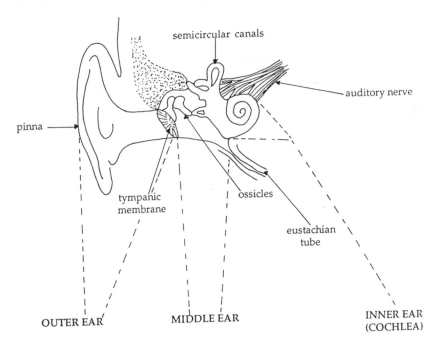

Figure 2.1 Diagram of the ear showing the outer, middle and inner ear, including the cochlea. Cochlear implants directly stimulate remaining auditory nerve fibres in the cochlea

usually permanent. Hearing loss caused by problems higher up the auditory pathway than the cochlea is described as neural. Sensory hearing impairments cannot be rectified surgically, but many sensory losses can be helped with conventional acoustic hearing aids which deliver an amplified signal into the ear canal. If, however, there is very little residual hearing, acoustic amplification will not give significant benefit. It is for these profoundly deaf patients that cochlear implantation may provide further access to audition. Cochlear implant systems electrically stimulate remaining auditory nerve tissue in the cochlea to induce a sensation of hearing. A comparison of the way in which acoustic hearing aids and cochlear implants function is shown in Figure 2.2. The benefits of cochlear implants for both adults and children have been well documented (Tyler, 1990; Cohen, Waltzman and Fisher, 1991; Miyamoto et al., 1991; Osberger et al.; 1991a). Profoundly deaf children implanted at a young age have been able to develop auditory/verbal communication with the aid of cochlear implants even though they have little or no experience of hearing (Hasenstab and Tobey, 1991; Osberger et al., 1991b; Tobey et al., 1991).

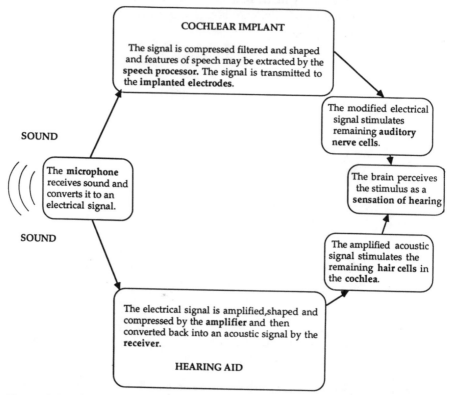

Figure 2.2 Differences in function of cochlear implants and conventional acoustic hearing aids

Historical development of cochlear implants

The early history of cochlear implantation has been recorded in some detail by Luxford and Brackmann (1985). Interest in the electrical stimulation of the cochlea has a long history, beginning with Volta's experiment in 1800, in which he stimulated his own ears electrically. The stimulation was unpleasant but produced some sound sensation. Considerably later, in 1930, Weaver and Bray discovered that the cochlea essentially acts as a transducer of acoustical energy into electrical energy, which is then transmitted via the auditory neural pathway to the brain. This provided further inspiration for the possibility of evoking artificial hearing through direct electrical stimulation. Djourno and Eyries (1957) first reported direct stimulation of the auditory nerve with an electric current. The subject described some auditory sensation which aided his lipreading ability and made him aware of background noise. There was, however, considerable doubt about the safety of the technique and its feasibility long term until new microsurgical procedures were developed. The first clinical cochlear implant was developed by Dr William House in the 1960s, after considerable research including electrical engineering input from Mr Jack Urban (House et al., 1976; House and Berliner, 1991). This first system was a relatively simple device using one active electrode, but over a period of years it gave significant benefit to implanted subjects. This implant was known as the House Implant and later the 3M/House Implant when the 3M company took over commercial production of the device. This implant system is no longer available.

During the time that House introduced the first clinical cochlear implant systems, research into electrical stimulation in the cochlea using multiple electrodes was being carried out by Simmons (1966). Advances in cardiac pacemakers in the 1950s and 1960s increased knowledge of biocompatible materials, insulation of electrodes and the effects of electrical stimulation which helped in cochlear implant research.

Interest in cochlear implantation had been stimulated by House, Urban and Simmons in the USA, but researchers have also been active in Europe and Australia. In France, Chouard (1980) developed multichannel systems; Hochmair, Hochmair-Desoyer and Burian worked on a multichannel device in Austria, but then changed to a simpler single-channel device which became commercially available and was known as the 3M/Vienna device (Burian, Hochmair-Desoyer and Elsenwort, 1986). In Australia, Dr Graeme Clark carried out extensive research developing a multichannel system with considerable emphasis on speech-processing strategies. This implant system also became commercially available and was originally known as the Nucleus Melbourne Cochlear Implant (Clark et al., 1987). Another multichannel system also became available following earlier research into multichannel stimulation in the USA. This device was known as the Symbion or Utah device and later the Ineraid cochlear implant (Eddington et al., 1978).

Research into cochlear implantation at the centres already mentioned and by other groups was now gathering pace; in fact it is still advancing rapidly. Many questions also arose during this period of rapid development, such as which candidates are suitable for implantation, which is the best type of implant system, what constitutes a successful implantee, how we can measure the survival of auditory nerve tissue and how safe is long-term electrical stimulation within the cochlea. The answers to these questions are continually evolving as knowledge increases further.

There has been resistance to implantation from the deaf community world wide who believe that hearing people are trying to 'cure' the deaf and their deafness. Cochlear implants should be regarded as a sophisticated type of hearing aid which offer another choice for help with communication for profoundly deaf individuals rather than a cure for deafness. Tyler (1993) has discussed cochlear implants and the deaf community in more depth, and ethical issues of paediatric cochlear implantation are addressed in Chapter 5. Although many researchers in the field of cochlear implantation felt that deaf children would have the greatest potential to gain most from cochlear implants, there was reluctance to proceed with implanting children until data had been gathered from implanted adults with acquired hearing losses.

As the evidence detailing the benefits of implantation for adults increased with few adverse effects, House decided to begin implanting children with his single-channel system. Most children received significant benefit from their implants (House, Berliner and Eisenberg, 1983), and the implantation of children became more widespread as the benefits of multichannel intracochlear stimulation became more evident. Thus, the Nucleus 22 Channel Implant, developed by Clark, has become the most widely used implant system in children. In the UK, cochlear implantation has been accepted slowly with the realisation that not everyone can receive benefit from conventional hearing aids, and in the light of the benefits of implantation documented in other countries. Cochlear implantation in the UK can no longer be considered as an experimental option even for children (Rosen, 1990; McCormick, 1991).

The development of cochlear implantation does not, however, comprise only the construction of the implant system itself; it also includes the evolution of methods to help optimise the use of the implant and facilitate implantees in learning to understand the new sound sensation they receive. In a survey by Tucci, Lambert and Ruth (1990), all clinicians polled agreed that rehabilitation was of great importance, and required more resources, in terms of time, for children to promote the successful use of implants. The process of implantation is therefore somewhat like obtaining a new computer. The hardware is useless without the software or proper programming, or setting up of the device; even with the correct 'software' the use of the computer or implant is greatly enhanced by appropriate written and verbal information and advice or rehabilitation. Most of this book is concerned with rehabilitation, but the purpose of this chapter is to describe the hardware and how it functions.

Components of a cochlear implant system

Cochlear implant systems are made up of several components and all require that the patient wears equipment externally as well as having an internal implanted electrode array. The external equipment consists of the microphone, the speech processor and a means of transferring the signal to the implanted electrodes (Figure 2.3).

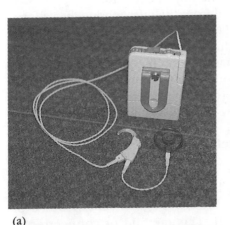

(a)

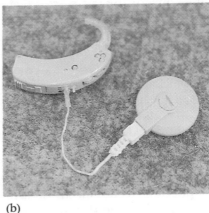

(b)

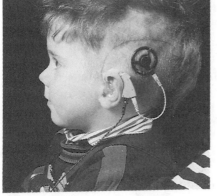

(c)

Figure 2.3 External components of cochlear implant systems: (a) the Nucleus bodyworn speech processor and headset; (b) the MedEl behind-the-ear speech processor and transmitter coil; and (c) a child using the Nucleus speech processor and headset

Microphone

The function of the microphone is to collect sound from the environment and convert it into an electrical signal. For most systems, the microphone is housed in its own case which is similar in shape, although slimmer, than a small postaural hearing aid. A lead transfers the electrical signal from the microphone to the speech processor. There is, however, now available one system with a postaural speech processor which has an integral microphone (Hochmair-Desoyer, Hochmair and Klasek, 1991) (Figure 2.3).

Speech processor

Apart from the system with the postaural processor mentioned above, the speech processor is body-worn, most using a belt clip or, for younger children, a harness. With body-worn processors there is no integral microphone so the processor can be worn under the clothing with no adverse effect on the quality of the signal. The speech processor contains the batteries to power the implant system. The processor also converts the raw electrical signal from the microphone into a form that can be delivered to the implanted electrode array. The speech processor either has an internal chip programmed by a computer or internal switches which are set manually by the audiologist. Speech processors have user-operated on/off, sensitivity and/or volume switches which affect the output of the processor and are discussed in more detail in Chapter 7.

Signal transfer to the implanted electrodes

The signal from the speech processor then needs to be delivered to the internal electrode array. This may be achieved by a direct hardware connection to the electrode array through the skin via a pedestal or plug fixed surgically into the skull. This method of connection is known as percutaneous. Where the skin is intact, an alternative transcutaneous connection may be used. An external transmitter sends the signal via an FM carrier wave to the internal receiver stimulator; here the signal is converted back into an electrical signal, stimulating the implanted electrodes. In most systems using transcutaneous links, the transmitter coil and internal receiver/stimulator are magnetised both to maintain a good contact across the skin and to keep the transmitter coil correctly aligned to the internal receiver.

Implanted electrode array

This comprises the implanted electrodes, which may be ring shaped or ball shaped, and the connection to the plug for percutaneous systems or the receiver/stimulator for transcutaneous systems. To induce an electrical field, current needs to flow from an active electrode or positive pole to a reference electrode or negative pole. There may be a separate reference electrode or this can be incorporated into the array of active electrodes. To maintain longevity the implant must be constructed to a very high standard and under clean conditions. The internal implant package is sealed within a biocompatible material, such as Silastic, to isolate it from body tissue and avoid any undesired non-auditory stimulation or tissue changes, and also to ensure that the implant is not affected by body fluids. Shepherd, Franz and Clark (1990) have addressed biocompatibility issues in detail with reference to the Nucleus 22 channel implant. The processed signal thus reaches the internal electrodes. The resultant electrical field stimulates the remaining auditory nerve fibres in the cochlea, and the signal is transmitted up the auditory neural pathway to the brain to give the implanted child a sensation of hearing.

Cochlear implant design

Cochlear implant systems all provide a means of detecting sound, processing the signal and conveying this electrical signal via implanted electrodes to remaining auditory nerve tissue. The design of the different implant systems does, however, vary in the number and position of electrodes, the processing of the incoming signal, and whether systems use transcutaneous or percutaneous transfer of information to the implanted electrodes.

Position of electrodes

Cochlear implants have been described as monopolar or bipolar according to the relative positions of the active and reference electrodes. In a monopolar system, the active and reference electrodes are positioned remotely, e.g. the active electrode may be inside the cochlea and the reference electrode embedded in muscle tissue outside the cochlea. If the active and reference electrodes are in close proximity, e.g. adjacent to each other inside the cochlea, the implant is known as a bipolar system. Current spreads over a wider area with monopolar systems than bipolar configurations which activate more discrete groups of neurons. Bipolar stimulation can be advantageous when information is sent to different groups of nerve fibres, but more current is required to produce the same level of stimulation with bipolar than with monopolar electrodes because fewer fibres are stimulated around the electrode.

The terms 'intracochlear' and 'extracochlear' are used to describe the site of the active electrodes of a cochlear implant. Extracochlear systems can be considered less invasive because the active electrode is placed outside the cochlea on the promontory or round window. Extracochlear electrodes are more distant from the auditory nerve tissue inside the cochlea and are, therefore, likely to require higher current levels. Intracochlear electrodes are inserted inside the cochlea which requires the surgeon to drill into, and therefore cause some damage to, the cochlea and any residual hearing (Boggess, Baker and Balkany, 1989). The loss of any residual hearing has to be balanced against the additional benefit which may be afforded by intracochlear multichannel stimulation. Less current is required with intracochlear systems and it may be possible to convey more complex information more effectively using an intracochlear system. Hortman et al. (1989) describe an extracochlear multichannel system, but this has not so far shown the same promise as intracochlear multichannel systems.

Single- and multichannel cochlear implants

The descriptions of single- or multi-electrode implants apply to the number of potentially active electrodes that the system has. The terms 'single-channel' and 'multichannel' have a different meaning and refer to the number of active electrodes through which different information is transmitted. A single-channel system may also be a single-electrode system, having one active electrode through which all the information is transmitted. Occasionally several electrodes are implanted, but only one electrode is selected to convey the signal (Hochmair, Hochmair and Zierhofer 1990) or the same information could be transmitted through several active electrodes. These types of system can be described as single-channel, multi-electrode. If several electrodes are implanted, usually inside the cochlea, and different information is conveyed through different electrodes, the device can be described as multichannel.

At the present time, the general consensus of opinion supports the view that intracochlear multichannel cochlear implants give rise to better patient performance than single-channel systems. The performance of single- and multichannel implantees has been studied using an extensive range of speech discrimination tasks (Cohen, Waltzman and Fisher, 1991, 1993). Although these authors obtained good results from single-channel users, the multichannel users made larger improvements over a wider range of tests, and there was no test in which the single-channel users out-performed the multichannel ones. Patients who have had single-channel implants replaced with multichannel devices have been shown to improve in tests of speech and environmental sound recognition (Doyle, Pijl and Noel, 1991). The degree of improvement did, however, vary considerably among different individual implantees. Parisier et al. (1991) found, in a series of patients re-implanted with multichannel devices after using single-channel ones, that the performance of most, but not all, implantees improved. In a case study in which a single-channel implant was replaced with a multi-channel ones in the same ear, there was improved performance with the multichannel device (Pijl, 1991). The speech and non-speech sounds uttered by children using single-channel implants have been compared to those using multichannel implants by video analysis techniques (Osberger et al., 1991c). The children using multichannel implants showed greater improvements in speech production than those using single-channel implants.

Research into single versus multichannel implants has to be viewed in the context that most report considerable variation among different subjects regardless of which device is being studied. In addition, many other factors may influence the implantees' performance, such as age and duration of deafness, nerve tissue survival and length of time of implant use. Studies have involved the small number of different types of implant system widely available which vary in their signal-processing strategies and other design features. Different multichannel devices have often been compared with the 3M/House single-channel device, which was widely used in the USA and the 3M/Vienna single-channel device. Just as there are differences among multichannel devices, different levels of performance have been recorded with different single-channel devices (Tyler, 1988). With the establishment of multichannel devices, further development of single-channel devices slowed down. Recently, however, new single-channel devices have become available in response to the demands of some, but not all, clinicians who wanted an alternative to multichannel intracochlear devices for implant candidates with ossified or deformed cochleas; this was the result of either difficulty in inserting multichannel devices in an ossified cochlea or possible increased risk of complications or potential programming difficulties for patients with deformed cochleas (Harnsberger et al., 1987; Balkany, Gantz and Nadol, 1988; Gray et al., 1991). Currently, most implant programmes would opt to use an intracochlear multichannel device as their first choice, although they may use an extracochlear single-channel device for particular patients. As more patients are implanted with different types of single- and multichannel devices, differences between the two types of system should become more apparent.

Speech-processing strategies

All implant systems use some form of processing of the raw signal from the microphone in the speech processor. Different philosophies in processing strategies have been applied to different implant systems. The processed signal may be delivered to the electrode array in different ways – as an analogue or continuous waveform or as a series of short fast pulses (pulsatile) representing a digitised sample of the original waveform.

Processing of the incoming sound signal is necessary to represent as fully as possible the acoustic signal in the narrow window available for electrical stimulation. This is the region between the level of electrical stimulation of the cochlea which first induces a hearing sensation and that level just below which electrical stimulation becomes uncomfortable. This is the dynamic range for electrical stimulation in a normally hearing ear which extends from very quiet background sound up to very loud levels, equivalent to the sound of jet engines, before sound becomes painful. Compression of the signal is therefore essential. Some filtering and frequency equalisation of the signal is also used to ensure that the signal waveform is evenly represented.

The goal of all cochlear implant speech-processing strategies is to give implantees some ability to discriminate speech auditorily. Different approaches have been employed in speech processors of different implant systems used clinically. Most single-channel devices such as the House (House et al., 1976), UCH/RNID (Cooper et al., 1989) and the Vienna (Hochmair-Desoyer et al., 1989) devices use a broad-band analogue signal which has been compressed, filtered and frequency equalised, and then delivered to a single active electrode. More recently some pulsatile single-channel devices have, however, been developed – the Monosonic by Chouard's group (Roulleau and Matha, 1989) and the Nucleus single-channel implant (Dillier, 1993).

The most widely used multichannel cochlear implants have been the Nucleus 22 channel cochlear implants (Clark et al., 1987) and the Ineraid (formerly Richards or Symbion) (Eddington et al., 1978) cochlear implant. Both systems use different signal-processing strategies. The Ineraid system has an array of six ball electrodes implanted inside the cochlea. The four electrodes with the best dynamic range are selected for stimulation. The system is analogue, and different frequency equalised bands of the filtered signal waveform are transmitted simultaneously. Different frequency bands of the filtered spectrum, i.e. different pitches, are delivered to each of the four channels, attempting to follow the tonotopic arrangement of the cochlea. The Nucleus 22 channel implant employs a different philosophy in speech processing to try to enhance the relatively important features of speech for discrimination, i.e. the fundamental frequency $F0$, the first formant $F1$ and the second formant $F2$. Early processing strategies for the Nucleus implant coded $F0$ as the rate of stimulation and $F2$ by place of stimulation along the electrode array, again mimicking the tonotopic arrangement of the cochlea. Further research resulted in a change in the processing strategy to $F0$, $F1$, $F2$ (Tye-Murray, Lowder and Tyler, 1990), which improved implantees' speech understanding. The wearable speech processor (WSP) for the Nucleus 22 system was superseded by the mini speech processor (MSP) and a newer processing strategy known as Multipeak was introduced which extracts $F0$, $F1$, $F2$, together with three high-frequency bands of information (von Wallenburg and Battmer, 1991).

The performance of implantees with Nucleus and Ineraid devices has been compared. Gantz et al. (1988) found similar levels of performance in discrimination tasks for both the Ineraid and Nucleus implantees in quiet conditions. In background noise the Ineraid implantees performed better than the Nucleus implantees, but at the time of this study the Nucleus implantees were using the $F0$, $F1$, $F2$ coding strategy. The introduction of the Multipeak coding strategy improved speech recognition in noise with the Nucleus implant (von Wallenberg and Battmer, 1991). A more recent study by Teig et al. (1992) compared the performance of Ineraid implantees with Nucleus implantees, using the MSP processor with the Multipeak coding strategy. Slightly better results were obtained from the Ineraid implantees, although the study only covered a small number of subjects and two of the Nucleus implantees were later found to have extensive nerve damage which would have influenced the results.

Tye-Murray et al. (1992) found similar development of discrimination skills in Ineraid and Nucleus implantees over an 18-month period after implantation. Thus two different approaches to processing the incoming signal with two quite different multichannel cochlear implants had both produced equally good results. The Ineraid device has used the compressed analogue form of signal processing which, because it is continuous and analogue, does not disrupt the timing clues in the signal waveform; however, by using simultaneous transmission to all four channels, there may be interactions between the channels producing unpredictable stimulation. Variations in pitch perception by Ineraid patients have been reported by Dorman et al. (1990). On the other hand, with the Nucleus device only one channel is stimulated at a time and stimulus pulses switch between electrodes so there should be no channel interactions. The pulsatile nature of the device and the feature-extraction processing will affect the timing clues in the speech signal. Thus the Nucleus system is relying on the pulse rate and stimulation of different electrodes, and therefore on different places in the cochlea to give different pitch percepts.

New developments in speech processing and implant systems

Research is ongoing into new speech-processing strategies. Wilson (1993) has discussed the results from more recent speech-processing strategies, including his own group's continuous interleaved sampling (CIS) strategy. Subjects implanted with the Ineraid implants were initially asked to use the new CIS strategy instead of their conventional compressed analogue Ineraid processors. The interchange was possible because the Ineraid implant has a direct hard wire connection through a percutaneous plug. All subjects showed improvements in their ability to discriminate speech even after short periods of use of the CIS system (Wilson et al., 1991). The CIS processing technique involves presenting different filtered sections of the signal waveform in short fast pulses, interleaving between electrodes at a very fast pulse rate. The filtered information is thus presented sequentially which should eliminate channel interactions. The very fast pulse rate such as 2500 pulses per second (p.p.s.) compared to the maximum possible pulse rate of 300–600 p.p.s. for the Nucleus device means that the timing clues in the signal are more likely to be conserved with the CIS strategy. Feature extraction is not employed by the CIS strategy.

Further work is continuing with the Nucleus device, including new processing strategies for the MSP, a new speech processor and new implants for specialised use. The latest processing strategy is the spectral maximum processing strategy (McKay et al., 1991) and involves selecting the six highest peaks from the speech frequency range and presenting this information at 250 p.p.s. to electrodes at positions along the electrode array on the basis of the spectral frequencies. This new processing strategy can be used in the new SPEAK processor, but it is still being evaluated. Early results show improvements over Nucleus processing strategies currently being used clinically. New implant designs of the Nucleus 20 +2 implant, which uses monopolar rather than bipolar stimulation modes, are being evaluated for particular patients (von Wallenberg et al., 1993).

New implant systems are also becoming available from other groups. In the USA, a new multichannel implant called the Clarion implant is undergoing clinical evaluation (Schindler and Kessler, 1992). This system has 16 channels and is a transcutaneous system; however, it is one that has the versatility for a wide range of signal-processing strategies to be used, including the CIS strategy. A multichannel device known as the Laura device is now available clinically. This device has 16 channels and also has considerable versatility, allowing high pulse rates and transcutaneous transmission (Peeters, Offeciers and Marquet, 1990). A new device being evaluated by the Vienna team uses an eight-channel multichannel implant with a combined analogue and pulsatile (CAP) speech-processing strategy (Hochmair-Desoyer, Hochmair and Klasek, 1991). Multichannel cochlear implants have been designed by the French group (Roulleau and Matha, 1989).

Some of the newer implant systems have the ability to carry out telemetry, i.e. test the impedance or function of internal electrodes. This facility is very useful in young children who may be unable to describe strange sound or non-sound sensations occurring when an electrode fails. It is also valuable to begin initial stimulation with the confidence of knowing which electrodes are functioning. The newer generation of cochlear implants, along with increased flexibility, bring increased complexity and more programming choice for the audiologist. More time may need to be spent programming more complex systems because it may be necessary to try a variety of options. The question of which programming strategy to start with also becomes a more complex issue.

There are too many implant systems in the early stages of development to cover in detail here. Mecklenburg and Lehnhardt (1991) list the main features of 38 devices at various stages of development and clinical use world wide excluding the USA. Lance de Foa and Loeb (1991) also list research and clinical uses of several different implant systems world wide. Thus, it is clear that there is a considerable degree of interest in cochlear implant systems and that the progress of development of new systems is rapid.

Choice of an implant system for children

When considering which cochlear implant systems to use with children, several factors need to be taken into account. Probably the two most important considerations for both adults and children are the safety of the device and the benefit afforded by it. Time is required to evaluate both safety and benefit which necessitates balancing the advantage of using newer more sophisticated devices against a device with a proven 'track record' for safety and benefit, although, perhaps, not giving the same potential as newer devices. It can be argued that children require higher levels of both safety and clarity from cochlear implants, because they are a more demanding population than adult implantees. Deaf children are implanted early in their lives and will, therefore, need to use their implants for considerably longer than many adult implantees. Young children being considered for implantation often have little or no memory of spoken language. They will therefore be learning a new language, albeit a second language for signers, rather than reawakening a language already known to adults with acquired hearing losses. Thus, although children are more adaptable to learning than adults, they may require a better signal from their implant if the ultimate goal is to develop speech and language auditorily.

Most implant teams select devices which have been widely and successfully used in adults before considering them for children. In the USA, the Food and Drug Administration (FDA) regulates trials of new cochlear implants and devices must have FDA approval before they can be used other than in a controlled research setting. The FDA therefore maintains tight control over the type of implant used; this can have the drawback of delaying the availability of new technology to candidates for implantation. The Nucleus device is currently the only implant available that has full FDA approval for use with children.

Cochlear implants are evolving rapidly and will undoubtedly allow better speech discrimination and speech production in the future. The question then arises as to whether children should be implanted at a young age or whether they should wait for a better device to become available. It has been reported that teenagers and adults deafened at an early age obtain less benefit from implantation than those implanted at a young age or after a relatively short duration of deafness (Parisier and Chute, 1991; Waltzman, Cohen and Shapiro, 1992). Although implantation with a different device is possible, it obviously involves further surgery. There is, however, support for early implantation of young children because little difference in terms of speech and language acquisition has been recorded between congenitally deaf children and those who acquired their hearing loss at a young age, both of whom were implanted at an early age. Both groups have obtained significant benefit (Osberger et al., 1991d). Parents need to be able to make well-informed decisions on behalf of their child about when and if to go ahead with implantation (Downs and Owen Black, 1985; Quittner, Thompson Steck and Rouiller, 1991). The benefits of cochlear implantation for children are, however, well documented (Osberger et al., 1991a; Staller et al., 1991; Gibbin, 1992).

Safety and longevity of cochlear implants are important considerations and are dependent on the design of implants, the quality of the components, and the quality and cleanliness of the manufacturing process. Issues of safety and biocompatibility have been discussed in detail elsewhere for different devices (House and Berliner, 1986; Shepherd, Franz and Clark, 1990). Complications and failure rates for different systems have also been reported (Cohen and Hoffman, 1991; Parisier and Chute, 1991) and should be taken into account bearing in mind the length of time and number of each particular device that has been implanted. Gersdorff (1991) reports a low complication rate following implantation of children which is no higher than that for adults.

Ergonomic features of cochlear implant systems can facilitate or hinder the child's use of the system. Although percutaneous plugs confer a technical advantage in that the system is more amenable to new processing strategies, transcutaneous systems do not have the disadvantage of complications arising from pedestal infections (Cohen and Hoffman, 1991). Children have, however, been successfully implanted with the Ineraid percutaneous system (Montandon, Kasper and Pelizzone, 1991), although most implant programmes for children use transcutaneous systems. The external equipment needs to be sufficiently small to be worn comfortably by children, but it also needs to be durable because young children are very active. Leads that can be unplugged are an advantage for children because they are often put under stress and breakage of a lead does not then require the replacement of the whole of the external equipment. A behind-the-ear processor would have one less lead which is susceptible to pulling and damage. Batteries are needed to power the external equipment and these should be easy to obtain. Rechargeable batteries are often available but may not last for a full day. This could be a disadvantage with a young child who may not consistently be able to indicate when the battery has gone flat. A low battery warning light on the processor is helpful for parents and teachers. The Nucleus implant system has a microphone light on the processor which flashes with auditory signals and a coil light which can be used to check that a signal is being transmitted through the coil. These features are reassuring for parents and teachers of young implanted children.

Once implanted, patients require good back-up from their implant centre, and also from the implant manufacturers in terms of providing replacement equipment and carrying out repairs. It is therefore important for the implant manufacturers to be financially secure and also be committed to existing patients. Different cochlear implants are not easily interchangeable in that surgery is required. In addition to maintaining the external equipment for existing patients, it would be advantageous if new processors or processing strategies could be designed so that existing as well as new implantees can benefit from them.

Once fitted with an implant system the aim is for the implantee to use the device as much as possible. For children in their educational setting, the same problems with background noise can occur for implantees as with conventional hearing aid users. In certain circumstances it would therefore be useful to be able to interface an FM radio aid with speech processors. A method of coupling the processor and radio receiver unit is needed and not all speech processors have this facility. The use of FM aids with speech processors is discussed further in Chapter 7. Ideally the cochlear implant should provide significant benefit to the patient without restricting his or her lifestyle. Obviously the wearing of the external equipment is a physical restriction in itself. Radio-frequency interference may restrict the use of the speech processor (Hocking, Joyner and Fleming, 1991). Medical investigations using magnetic resonance imaging cannot be used with most types of cochlear implant because of the torsion created by the strong magnetic field involved (Portnoy and Mattucci, 1991). Medical considerations regarding implantation are discussed further in Chapter 5. It is important that implant candidates and their families are aware of any possible restrictions that may be experienced as a result of implantation.

The factors affecting the choice of implant systems for children are summarised in Table 2.1. Programmes may opt to choose more than one system, e.g. the preferred choice for a patent, normally formed cochlea may be a multichannel device but for children with an ossified or malformed cochlea an extracochlear single-channel device may be preferred. The Nucleus 22 channel cochlear implant has been the most widely used system in children to date, perhaps because it has been

Table 2.1 Factors affecting the choice of an implant system for children

Essential requirements	*Additional considerations*
Device safety	Percutaneous versus transcutaneous
Proven benefit	transmission
Back-up for equipment	Single versus multichannel
spares and repairs	Type of processing strategy
	Durability of the implant system and ease of changing the external components of the system
	Size of external equipment
	Availability of batteries and length of battery life
	Lights on the processor to indicate battery charge and that a signal is being transmitted
	Possibility of interfacing the implant device with an FM system

judged to meet the most requirements for an implant for children at the present time.

Conclusion

Cochlear implantation has progressed rapidly since House's first clinical cochlear implant system. Research into cochlear implantation has progressed from the development of the first single-channel device to very sophisticated and flexible multichannel devices which offer great potential benefit to profoundly and severely hearing-impaired adults and children. Only adults were implanted initially, followed by children with acquired hearing losses and then young congenitally deaf children. It is now clear that all these groups can obtain significant benefit from implantation. In the future it is likely that there may be more children implanted than adults and that newer devices and processing strategies, currently being evaluated with adults, will become available for children. The field of cochlear implantation has developed from its infancy to its adolescence. There will no doubt be further advances in signal-processing strategies, miniaturisation and design of cochlear implant systems over the next few years.

References

Balkany, T., Gantz, B. and Nadol, J.B. (1988). Multichannel cochlear implants in partially ossified cochleas. *Annals of Otology, Rhinology and Laryngology* **97**, 3–7.

Boggess, W.J., Baker, J.E. and Balkany, T.J. (1989). Loss of residual hearing after cochlear implantation. *The Laryngoscope* 99, 1002–1005.

Burian, K., Hochmair-Desoyer, I.J. and Eisenwort, B. (1986). The Vienna cochlear implant programme. *Otolaryngology Clinics of North America* 19, 313–328.

Chouard, C.H. (1980). The surgical rehabilitation of total deafness with the multichannel cochlear implant – indication and results. *Audiology* 19, 137–145.

Clark, G.M., Blamey, P.J., Brown, A.M., Gusby, P.A., Dowell, R.C., Franz, B. K-H., Pyman, B.C., Shepherd, R.K., Tong, Y.C., Webb, R.L., Hirshorn, M.S., Kuzma, J., Mecklenburg, D.J., Money, D.K., Patrick, J.F. and Seligman, P.M. (1987). The University of Melbourne–Nucleus multichannel cochlear implant In: C.R. Pfaltz (ed.), *Advances in Otology-Rhinology–Laryngology*, vol. 38. Basel: Karger.

Cohen, N.L. and Hoffman, R.A. (1991). Complications of cochlear implant surgery in adults and children. *Annals of Otology, Rhinology, Laryngology* 100, 708–711.

Cohen, N.L., Waltzman, S.B. and Fisher, S.G. (1991). Prospective randomized clinical trial of advanced cochlear implants. Preliminary results of a department of veterans affairs cooperative study. *Annals of Otology, Rhinology, Laryngology* 100, 823–829.

Cohen, N.L., Waltzman, S.B. and Fisher, S.G. (1993). A prospective randomized study of cochlear implants. *New England Journal of Medicine* 328, 233–237.

Cooper, H.R., Carpenter, L., Alesky, W., Booth, C.L., Read, T.E., Graham, J. M. and Fraser, J.G. (1989). UCH/RNID single channel extracochlear implant results in 30 profoundly deafened adults. *The Journal of Laryngology and Otology* 18 (Suppl.), 22–38.

Dillier, N. (1993). Initial results with Single Channel Encoders for the Nucleus MSP. Paper presented at the Cochlear Technical Workshop, Schönried, Switzerland, April 14–16 1993.

Djourno, A. and Eyries, C. (1957). Prostheses auditive par excitation electrique a distance du nerf sensoriel a l'aide d'un bobinage inclus a demeure. *Presse Medicale* 35, 14–17.

Dorman, M.F., Smith, L., McCandless, G., Dunnervant, G., Parkin, J. and Dankonski, K. (1990). Pitch scaling and speech understanding by patients who use the Ineraid Cochlear Implant. *Ear and Hearing* 11, 310–315.

Downs, M.P. and Owen Black, F. (1985). Cochlear implants for children: Counselling the parents. *Seminars in Hearing* 6 (1), 91–95.

Doyle, P.J., Pijl, S. and Noel, F.J. (1991). The cochlear implant: a comparison of single and multichannel results *Journal of Otolaryngology* 20, 204–208.

Eddington, D.K., Dobelle, W.H., Brackmann, E.E., Mladejousky, M.G. and Parkin, J.L. (1978). Auditory prosthesis research with multiple channel intracochlear stimulation in man. *Annals of Otology, Rhinology, Laryngology* 87 (Suppl. 53), 1–39.

Gantz, B., Tyler, R.S., Knutson, J.F., Woodworth, G., Abbas, P., McCabe, B. F., Hinrichs, J., Tye-Murray, N., Lansing, C., Kuk, F. and Brown, C. (1988). Evaluation of 5 different cochlear implant designs: audiological assessment and predictors of performance. *The Laryngoscope* 98, 1100–1106.

Gersdorff, M. (1991). Results of cochlear implants in children. *Acta Otol-Rhinol-Laryngologica Belgica*, 45, 293–295.

Gibbin, K.P. (1992). Paediatric cochlear implantation. *Archives of Disease in Childhood* 67, 669–671.

Gray, R., Evans, R.A., Freer, C.E.L., Szutowicz, H.E. and Maskell, G.F. (1991). Radiology for cochlear implants. *Journal of Laryngology and Otology* 105, 85–88.

Harnsberger, H. Ric., Dart, D.J., Parkin, J.L., Smoker, W.R.K. and Osborn, A.G. (1987). Cochlear implant candidates: Assessments with CT and MR Imaging. *Radiology* **164**, 53–57.

Hasenstab, S.M. and Tobey, E.A. (1991). Language development in children receiving Nucleus multichannel cochlear implants. *Ear and Hearing* **12** (Suppl. 4) 5S–65S.

Hochmair, E.S., Hochmair, I.J. and Zierhofer, C. (1990). Electronic circuits for cochlear implants. *Archiv für Elecktronic und Übertagungstechnik (Electronics and Communication)* **44**, 238–246.

Hochmair-Desoyer, I.J., Hochmair, E.S. and Klasek, O. (1991). New Vienna Cochlear Implant with postaural processor: Results. Presentation at the Annual Conference of the German HNO Company, May 1991, Aachen.

Hochmair-Desoyer, I.J., Hochmair, E.S., Zierhofer, C. and Stiglbrunner, H. (1989). A family of extra and intracochlear implant systems. *Proceedings of the International Symposium on 'Acquisitions and controversies in cochlear implants'*, Toulouse, pp. 361–372.

Hocking, B., Joyner, K.H. and Fleming, A.H.J. (1991). Implanted medical devices in workers exposed to radio-frequency radiation. *Scandinavian Journal of Work and Environmental Health* **17**, 1–6.

Hortman, G., Pulec, J.L., Causse, J.B., Causse, J.R., Briand, C., Fontaine, J.P., Tetu, F. and Azema, B. (1989). Experience with the extracochlear multichannel Implex system. In B. Fraysse (ed.), *Cochlear Implant Acquisitions and Controversies*, pp. 307–317. Basel: Cochlear. Manuscript of International Symposium, Toulouse, June 9–10 1989.

House, W.F., Berliner, K., Crary, W., Graham, M., Luckey, R., Norton, N., Selters, W., Tobin, H., Urban J. and Wexler, M. (1976). Cochlear implants. *Annals of Otology, Rhinology, Laryngology* **85** (Suppl. 27), 1–93.

House, W.F. and Berliner, K.I. (1986). Safety and efficacy of the House/3M cochlear implant in profoundly deaf adults. *Otolaryngology Clinics of North America* **19**, 275–286.

House, W.F. and Berliner, K.I. (1991). Cochlear implants: From idea to clinical practice. In H. Cooper (ed.), *Cochlear Implants: A Practical Guide*, pp. 9–33. London: Whurr.

House, W.F., Berliner, K.I. and Eisenberg, L.S. (1983). Experiences with the cochlear implant on preschool children. *Annals of Otology, Rhinology, Laryngology* **92**, 587–592.

Lance de Foa, J. and Loeb, G.E. (1991). Issues in cochlear prosthetics from an international survey of opinions. *International Journal of Technology Assessment in Health Care* **7**, 403–410.

Luxford, W.M. and Brackmann, D.E. (1985). The history of cochlear implants. In R. Gray (ed.), *Cochlear Implants*, pp. 1–26. London: Croom Helm.

McCormick, B. (1991). Paediatric cochlear implantation in the United Kingdom – a delayed journey on a well marked route. *British Journal of Audiology* **25**, 145–149.

McKay, C., McDermott, H., Vandali, A. and Clark, G. (1991). Preliminary results with a six spectral maxima sound processor for the University of Melbourne/Nucleus multiple electrode cochlear implant. *Journal of the Otolaryngology Society of Australia* **6** (5), 354–359.

Mecklenburg, D. and Lehnhardt, E. (1991). The development of cochlear implants in Europe, Asia and Australia', In Cooper H. (ed.), *Cochlear Implants: A Practical Guide*, pp. 34–57. London: Whurr.

Miyamoto, R.T., Osberger, M.J., Robbins, A.M., Myres, W.A., Kessler, K. and Pope, M.L. (1991). Comparison of speech perception abilities in deaf children with hearing aids or cochlear implants. *Otolaryngology, Head and Neck Surgery* **104**, 42–46.

Montandon, P., Kasper, A. and Pelizzone, M. (1991). A case study of a 4 year old perilingually deaf child implanted with an Ineraid multichannel cochlear implant. *Otorhinolaryngology* **53**, 315–318.

Osberger, M.J., Miyamoto, R.T., Zimmerman-Phillips, S., Kemink, J.L., Stroer, B.S., Firszt, J.B. and Novak, M.A. (1991a). Independent evaluation of the speech perception abilities of children with the Nucleus 22 channel cochlear implant system. *Ear and Hearing* **12** (Suppl. 4) 66S–80S.

Osberger, M.J., Robbins, A.M., Miyamoto, R.T., Berry, S.W., Myres, W.A., Kessler, K.S. and Pope, M.L. (1991b). Speech perception abilities of children with cochlear implants, tactile aids or hearing aids. *American Journal of Otology* **12** (Suppl.) 105–115.

Osberger, M.J., Robbins, A.M., Berry, S.W., Todd, S.L., Hesketh, L.J. and Sedley, A. (1991c). Analysis of the spontaneous speech samples of children with cochlear implants or tactile aids. *American Journal of Otology* **12** (Suppl.), 151–164.

Osberger, M.J., Todd, S.L., Robbins, A.M., Berry, S.W. and Miyamoto, R.T. (1991d). Effect of age of onset of deafness on children's speech perception abilities with a cochlear implant. *Annals of Otology, Rhinology and Laryngology* **100**, 883–888.

Parisier, S. and Chute, P. (1991). Cochlear implants: Indications and technology. *Medical Clinics of North America* **75**, 1267–1275.

Parisier, S.C., Chute, P.M., Weiss, M.H., Hellman, S.A. and Wang, R.C. (1991). Results of cochlear implant reinsertion. *The Laryngoscope* **101**, 1013–1015.

Peeters, S., Offeciers, F.E. and Marquet, J.F.E. (1990). The Laura cochlear prothesis: technical aspects. In T. Sacriotan, J.J. Alvares-Vicent, J. Bartual et al. (eds), *Otorhinolaryngology, Head and Neck Surgery*, pp. 1193–1202. Proceedings of the XIV World Congress of Otorhinolaryngology, Head and Neck Surgery, Madrid, Spain 1989. Amsterdam: Kugler & Ghedini.

Pijl, S. (1991). Single-channel versus bilateral multichannel cochlear implant results: a case report. *Ear and Hearing* **12**, 431–433

Portnoy, W.M. and Mattucci K. (1991). Cochlear implants as a contraindication to magnetic resonance imaging. *Annals of Otology, Rhinology, Laryngology* **100**, 195–197.

Quittner, A.L., Thompson Steck, J. and Rouiller, R. (1991). Cochlear implants in children: a study of parental stress and adjustment. *American Journal of Otology* **12** (Suppl.), 95–104.

Rosen, S. (1990). Cochlear implants: some consensus at last?. *British Journal of Audiology* **24**, 361–373.

Roulleau, P. and Matha, N. (1989). Comparative Evaluation of performances obtained with Multi and Monochannel implants. A study of 40 patients. In B. Frassye (ed.), *Cochlear Implants – Acquisitions and Controversies*, pp. 417–426. Toulouse: Paragraphic.

Schindler, R.A. and Kessler, D.K. (1992). Preliminary results with the Clarion cochlear implant. *The Laryngoscope* **102**, 1006–1013.

Simmons, F.B. (1966). Electrical stimulation of the auditory nerve in man. *Archives of Otolaryngology*, **84**, 2–54.

Shepherd, R.K., Franz, B.K. - H.G. and Clark, G. (1990). The biocompatibility and safety of cochlear protheses. In G. Clark, Y.C. Tong and J.F. Patrick (eds),

Cochlear Prostheses pp. 69–98. London: Churchill Livingstone.

Staller, S., Beiter, A.L., Brimacombe, J.A., Mecklenburg, D.J. and Arnolt, P. (1991). Paediatric performance with the Nucleus 22 channel cochlear implant system. *The American Journal of Otology* 12 (Suppl.), 126–136.

Teig, E., Lindeman, H.H., Floltorp, G., Tvete, O., Hanche-Olson, S. and Arntsen, O. (1992). Patient performance with two types of multiple electrode intracochlear implants. *Scandinavian Audiology* 21, 93–99.

Tobey, E.A., Angelette, S., Murchison, C., Nicosia, J., Sprague, S., Staller, S., Brimacombe, J.A. and Beiter, A.L. (1991). Speech production performance in children with multichannel cochlear implants. *American Journal of Otology* 12 (Suppl.), 165–173.

Tucci, D.L., Lambert, P.R. and Ruth, R.A. (1990). Trends in rehabilitation after cochlear implantation. *Archives of Otolaryngology, Head and Neck Surgery* 116, 571–574.

Tye-Murray, N., Lowder, M. and Tyler, R.S. (1990). Comparison of the F0F2 and F0F1F2 Processing strategies for the Cochlear Corporation Cochlear Implant. *Ear and Hearing* 11, (3), 195–200.

Tye-Murray, N., Tyler, R.S., Woodworth, G.G. and Gantz, B.J. (1992). Performance over time with a Nucleus or Ineraid cochlear implant. *Ear and Hearing* 13 (3), 200–209.

Tyler, R.S. (1988). Open set word recognition with the 3M/Vienna single channel cochlear implant. *Archives of Otolarnygology, Head and Neck Surgery* 114, 1123–1126.

Tyler, R.S. (1990). Speech perception with the Nucleus cochlear implant in children trained with the auditory/verbal approach. *American Journal of Otology* 11, 99–107.

Tyler, R.S. (1993). Cochlear implants and deaf culture. *American Journal of Audiology* March, 26–32.

von Wallenberg, E.L. and Battmer, R.D. (1991). Comparative speech recognition results in eight subjects using two different coding strategies with the Nucleus 22 channel cochlear implant. *British Journal of Audiology* 25, 371–380.

von Wallenberg, E.L., Laszig, R., Gnadeberg, D., Battmer, R.D., Desloovere, C., Lehnhardt, E. and von Ilberg, C. (1993). Initial findings with a modified Nucleus Implant comprised of 20 active intracochlear and 2 extracochlear reference electrodes. Proceedings of the 3rd International Cochlear Implant Conference, Innsbruck, Austria, in press.

Waltzman, S.B., Cohen, N.L. and Shapiro, W.H. (1992). Use of a multichannel cochlear implant in the congenital and prelingually deaf population. *The Laryngoscope* 102, 395–399.

Wilson, B.S., Finley, C.C., Lawson, D.T., Wolford, R.D., Eddington, D.K. and Rabinowitz, W.M. (1991). Better speech recognition with cochlear implants. *Nature* 352 (18), 236–238.

Wilson, B.S. (1993). Signal processing. In R.S. Tyler (ed.), *Cochlear Implants: Audiological Foundations*, pp. 35–86. London: Whurr.

Chapter 3
Implementing a paediatric cochlear implant programme: theory and practice

SUE ARCHBOLD

This chapter considers the rationale for the development of a specialist paediatric cochlear implant programme, and its practical implementation, as an example of what may be required. Such a programme is described, emphasising the interface between the implant clinic and the professionals supporting the child at home and school. It gives protocols which have been adopted for the assessment, implantation, rehabilitation and maintenance phases; finally, it considers the staffing and long-term cost implications of such a programme.

Introduction

With encouraging results from cochlear implantation in deafened adults, implant teams throughout the world turned their attention to profoundly deaf children, amid much controversy. Children had received a single-channel implant at the House Ear Institute, Los Angeles, as early as 1980 and the first young child, aged 5, was implanted with the Nucleus 22 channel device, now the most commonly used in children, in Melbourne in 1986 (Mecklenburg, Demorest and Staller, 1991). Cochlear Corporation established the clinical trials necessary in the USA to obtain approval of the FDA (Food and Drug Administration) for implantation in children aged 2–17 years; this was obtained in 1990, by which time 600 children had received the device in this age group world wide.

For many years paediatric implantation, particularly in the case of congenitally deaf children, has been opposed by some of the groups involved with deaf children and adults. The controversy led to an unfortunate polarisation of views and delayed the development of a rational approach to implantation in which parents could make an informed decision on behalf of their child (McCormick, 1991). At the time of writing, controversy continues in Europe, Australia and the USA. It has not always been understood that implantation in a child involves broader issues than implantation in a deafened adult, and this chapter will consider some of these issues; many are not new in the management of deaf children but are familiar to those with experience of hearing-aided children.

An understanding of the deaf culture is often limited among professionals working with deaf children (Tyler, 1993a) and the views of deaf people about cochlear implantation have often not been explored fully by implant teams. Those who view themselves as members of the deaf community do not see deafness as a medical condition requiring treatment, but as a linguistic and cultural identity or social condition (Power and Hyde, 1992). Cochlear implantation may be seen as a threat to this identity, and as an attempt to effect a 'cure' (Cayton, 1991; Lea, 1991; Tyler, 1993a). Much of the publicity which has accompanied implantation and the use of terms such as 'bionic ear' promote this myth (Power and Hyde, 1992; Laurenzi, 1993). Cochlear implantation in children is not merely an audiological or medical process but one which, in providing useful audition to those previously unable to benefit from conventional aids, will affect a child's relationships with others, educational and communication options, and self-image as a deaf person. It is vital that those professionals involved in paediatric implantation become familiar with the issues associated with deafness, and ensure that parents of implant candidates also consider them, so that they can make an informed decision about implantation and understand the implications of their decision for their child's future.

Although there was initially a strong recommendation that paediatric implantation should only be carried out in those centres with experience of adult implantation, it is now increasingly recognised that a great deal of paediatric experience is necessary on the part of a wide range of professionals to carry out the assessment, implantation, tuning and rehabilitation of appropriate children (Fraser, 1991; Goin and Parisier, 1991; Kileny, Kemink and Zimmerman-Phillips, 1991) Professionals already involved in adult implantation may not possess the necessary expertise to deal with the issues involved with young, profoundly deaf children who have few communication skills. When establishing the Nottingham, UK team (McCormick, 1991; Archbold, 1992), it was considered more important to establish a specialist implant team with extensive relevant paediatric experience than to add a paediatric programme to an already established adult implant programme. What was the rationale behind the development of a specialist paediatric cochlear implant team?

Rationale for a specialist paediatric cochlear implant team

With deafened adults, the aim of implantation is to restore a channel of audition to facilitate communication in one who has already established language skills. With children born deaf or deafened at an early age, we are aiming for more than this: we are aiming to provide audition, as a means of developing basic spoken language skills. What factors can influence the achievement of this?

Kirk and Hill-Brown (1985) give a useful summary of published works on the adverse effects of profound hearing loss on the development of spoken language, explaining the influence of age at onset and degree of loss in predicting the severity of effect. The primary channel through which communication skills and thus spoken language are usually acquired is hearing; profound hearing loss can have a devastating effect on a child's linguistic development (Quigley and Kretschmer, 1984; Webster, 1986; Wood et al., 1986) and the resulting poor educational achievements are also well documented (Conrad, 1979; Wood et al., 1986). There are many complex influences on a deaf child's progress, but the degree of hearing loss is critical (Quigley and Kretschmer, 1984; Bamford and Saunders, 1991).

Children born deaf, or deafened at an early age, with a total, or near-total, hearing loss will be unable to acquire language through the channel of hearing and will be dependent upon a visual mode of communication, whether this is sign language, lipreading or the written form. Controversy has raged for over 100 years about the relative merits of oral/aural or sign-language approaches for deaf children. Acquisition of language by a sign-language approach, whether by spoken language supported by sign or a sign language with its separate grammar, may well have been more appropriate for a child audiologically suitable for implantation (Kessler and Owens, 1989).

Early amplification has been a desired goal for deaf children, but for some children conventional hearing aids will provide little benefit or little auditory access to speech. This is a small group of children (Geers and Moog, 1991; McCormick, 1991; Gibbin, 1992), but one for whom a cochlear implant can provide useful hearing. The age group 2–4 years is the most rapidly expanding group to be implanted, and this is the group which will demand the greatest expertise on the part of the implant team. These children are unlikely to have developed age-appropriate communication skills, are likely to be difficult to test audiologically and, should implantation take place, are unlikely to show immediate postoperative benefit (Somers, 1991). Although age at onset, length of deafness and communication mode have all been considered as predictors of positive outcomes from implantation, there is still little consensus of opinion on criteria for paediatric implantation (Osberger et al., 1991); indeed, the greater variability in outcome measures in children (Osberger, 1990) make candidate selection and prediction of benefit accordingly more difficult than in the adult population.

Although difficult to assess, two of the most important factors in enabling the effective use of a cochlear implant system may well be parental support and educational management. Family responsibilities will be discussed more fully later in the chapter, but there is also a growing acknowledgement of the influence of family expectations and the family's right and obligation to make the decision regarding this elective operation for their child, having considered the long-term implications and explored other management options. For children with conventional hearing aids, educational management, regardless of communication strategy, is a vital factor in influencing educational achievements (Wood et al., 1986; Boothroyd, 1989) and this is likely to be true for those with cochlear implants. The role of the child's educational management is emphasised by those with paediatric experience (Beiter, Staller and Dowell, 1991; Geers and Moog, 1991); the major ongoing support for the child post-implantation will be provided in the child's educational setting.

Experience is revealing an increased awareness on behalf of implanting surgeons (Fraser, 1991; Goin and Parisier, 1991; Gibbin, 1992; O'Donoghue, 1992) of these additional complexities of child implantation, which can be summarised as follows:

- The greater variability in outcome as opposed to that in the adult population.
- The correspondingly greater difficulty in pre-implant assessment and prediction of benefit.
- The number of variables influencing benefits: age of onset, aetiology, length of deafness, parental influence, educational management.
- The greater length of time taken to show benefit.
- The long-term commitment needed to be given to these children by the implant team.
- The role of parental responsibility in the decision-making process, and long-term parental commitment necessary.
- The wide range of professionals required to work together as a team, often based in different geographical centres.
- The more time-consuming nature of paediatric implantation.

Any paediatric implant team should consider these issues and the way in which they will meet the particular needs of the child, family and local professionals involved with the child; these influences on the team are illustrated in Figure 3.1.

The structure of a paediatric cochlear implant team

Having established the importance of the influences and responsibilities of parents and local educators, it is necessary to consider the cochlear implant team in its widest sense, including the 'team' at the

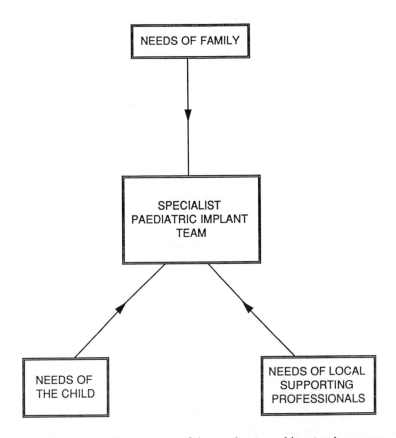

Figure 3.1 Influences on the structure of the paediatric cochlear implant team

child's home as well as the conventional cochlear implant team at the clinic. Figure 3.2 illustrates an example of a comprehensive paediatric implant team, including the local team at the child's home and the team at the implant clinic, with the child placed to indicate the central position in the process of implantation. In other countries, or at other implant centres, the professional responsibilities of members of staff and their titles may differ, but the overall expertise needed by the team will remain the same.

An element of mystique has built up about cochlear implantation and the programmes used to carry it out; the most vital personnel, however, may well be those working with the deaf child, whether implantation proceeds or not – the local team at the child's home.

The local team at the child's home

The child

The most important member of any implant team is not any of the

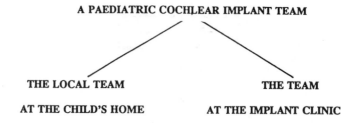

A PAEDIATRIC COCHLEAR IMPLANT TEAM

THE LOCAL TEAM   THE TEAM

AT THE CHILD'S HOME   AT THE IMPLANT CLINIC

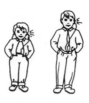

Parents	Coordinator/Administrator
Family	Surgeon
ENT Consultant	Nursing Staff
Audiological Scientist	Paediatric Audiological Scientist
Teacher of the Deaf	Medical Physicist
Other Educators	Teacher of the Deaf
Speech and Language Therapist	Speech and Language Therapist
Educational Psychologist	Educational Psychologist
Social Worker for the Deaf	Social Worker for the Deaf
Other carers	Technician

Figure 3.2 A paediatric cochlear implant team

professionals, but the child him- or herself. The child and his or her long-term needs must be the focus of any cochlear implant programme; as Staller, Beiter and Brimacombe (1991) state, paediatric implantation 'creates a life-long relationship between the implant team and the patient'. So that productive relationships can be established between the child and the implant clinic, a member of the clinic team, usually the implant clinic teacher of the deaf, must meet the child on his or her own ground – at school or nursery, and at home. Close observation of the child in a familiar setting will help assess the child's suitability for implantation, and establish baselines of functioning.

Children with no spoken language skills must be fully involved during the assessment period; they need to become familiar with the personnel at the implant clinic, and be prepared as fully as possible for implantation and future rehabilitation. Parents are usually the best guides as to their child's probable needs for preparation, which may depend on linguistic functioning; in Chapter 12 parents describe their experiences of preparing children for operation. The use of videos, photographs and colouring books may be helpful, together with contact with other children wearing the device (Downs, 1986). Older children need to be given explanations for the operation and some reasonable expectations; it can be difficult to balance giving an explanation with the possibility of raising the child's expectations falsely. If good relations have been established with the child and family from the outset, then it should prove possible to prepare the child appropriately, and to establish a basis for the 'life-long relationships' which may follow implantation.

The family

Deafness in one member of the family affects the others (Luterman, 1987) and cochlear implantation also does not affect merely the recipient. The needs of other members of the family must be considered and balanced in meeting the needs of the child receiving the cochlear implant; all too often, the needs of siblings may be overlooked as the family prepare the deaf child for implantation. Cochlear implantation and the rehabilitation period can be stressful for the whole family (Downs, 1986) and the support of other relatives will be vital for parents during the operative period, and the ensuing tuning and rehabilitation. Travelling long distances to the implant centre, as often occurs, will require the support of the family so that the effects on the other members are minimised.

Studies by Quittner, Thompson Steck and Rouiller (1991) show high levels of stress in parents of hearing-impaired children before and after implantation, as some of the parental comments in Chapter 12 illustrate. Levels of parental responsibility are high and counselling towards realistic expectations must include the whole family. If early benefit is not seen following implantation (as is probable with young children), disappointment expressed by other members of the family is most unhelpful. Similarly, if expected benefits are not observed then the child must not feel responsible and parents must remain supportive (Evans, 1989). Grandparents are often a useful source of support for parents of deaf children (Luterman, 1987) and, if they have been involved during the preparation period by inclusion in visits and the loan of information materials, their support is likely to be realistic during the postoperative phase.

Parents, however, remain the strongest source of support for their child (Evans, 1989). Contact with other parents has been found to promote greater understanding of the probable difficulties and an arena for sharing feelings which is not possible with implant professionals; this is the factor that is mentioned most frequently as helping parents before implantation (see Chapter 12). The implant clinic bears some responsibility for facilitating this contact; several teams have active parents' support groups and newsletters. An international support newsletter, has now been in existence for 3 years (TUNE-INternational, edited by S. Archbold and available from Cochlear UK) and has proved a well-used means of sharing the responsibilities of cochlear implantation.

The child's local teachers: mainstream and specialist

The postoperative management of the child will fall largely on the teacher in the child's educational setting (Geers and Moog, 1991; Goin and Parisier, 1991; Somers, 1991); in addition, this teacher will provide long-term support for the family (Osberger et al., 1991). With young children this can be a qualified teacher of the deaf visiting at home or in a nursery setting; this can also be a non-specialist teacher working in a mainstream class receiving support from a visiting teacher of the deaf. Whatever the child's educational setting, teaching staff must be involved from the beginning in the assessment of the suitability of the child and in the discussion of the child's long-term rehabilitation needs if implantation proceeds. The child's local teacher of the deaf will see the child on a more regular basis than the implant clinic teacher; this teacher brings insights into the child's everyday functioning and a knowledge of the local educational options for that child which are invaluable to the implant team. Establishing the cooperation of the child's educational support staff for the ongoing rehabilitation of a child will involve assessment of the communication and educational management styles in operation, as well as practical issues such as the suitability of the acoustical environment for developing listening skills.

Peer group preparation is also important; the peer group can be a strong influence on the long-term acceptance of the device, and local teachers can help the other children (deaf and/or hearing) and their parents to understand what cochlear implantation will involve and why it was necessary. Cochlear implantation in one of their pupils may well raise many questions for other children in their care; teachers of the deaf must be well informed to explain which children may, or may not, be suitable.

Local speech and language therapists

In the UK, the amount and type of speech and language therapy offered to hearing-impaired children varies widely; its availability must be encouraged by the implant team and, as with the local teacher of the deaf, close cooperation must be established from the outset between the implant team speech and language therapists and the local therapist.

Examples of this cooperation are given in Chapter 11. Assessments before and after implantation must be made in collaboration with the local therapist, as well as the educator, and future rehabilitation and assessment planned jointly.

Local audiological scientist

The child's local audiological scientist may have been closely involved in the audiological management of the child before implantation; after implantation, there may be little that the audiological scientist can do beyond simple trouble-shooting of the system, as a result of the complex programming equipment required for most devices. The provision of spares, replacements and repairs will usually be managed by the implant centre, as will tuning of the device and monitoring of the system. An interested audiologist may find it difficult to have little professional responsibility, and the implant centre should involve the child's scientist where possible, through organised visits and regular reports.

Local ENT consultants

In the UK, the referral to the implant centre will generally be made by the child's local ENT consultant or audiological physician, and the implant surgeon may well need to consult with the local specialists about medical and surgical assessments. When the child lives at some distance from the implant centre, the local consultant should be asked to cooperate in the postoperative care and long-term medical support of the child. Parents find it reassuring to know that local medical support and cooperation has been established between the implanting surgeon and local otolaryngologist before implantation.

Local educational psychologist

Most hearing-impaired children in the UK will have an educational psychologist responsible for ensuring that a statutory Statement of Special Educational Needs (SEN) is completed as appropriate, outlining their special educational needs and ensuring that these needs are met. This is equivalent to the IEP (Individualized Education Plan) in the USA. During the assessment period, contact should be made with the local psychologist to ask for a contribution to the child's assessment. It is important that all areas of a child's development are explored, because any other learning difficulties may influence rehabilitation and the probable benefits from the implant system. A cochlear implant may well influence future educational placement, and an educational psychologist who shares the responsibility for the decisions made about educational choices for the child must have realistic expectations of implantation.

Local social worker for the deaf

Any social worker for the deaf appointed to the child and family must be involved in the assessment of a child for implantation. In practice, in the UK, comparatively few deaf children have an assigned social worker for the deaf, but where a social worker – generic or specialist – is supporting the child and family, that person must share in the preparation period and also be made aware of the implications of implantation. A social worker for the deaf will often be in contact with the local deaf community and have insights into the deaf culture which are useful to the family considering implantation. This contact, if available, is an important one for the clinic team to develop, to strengthen understanding about implantation within the deaf community and to overcome the problems of misinformation among deaf people.

Other carers

Deaf children are the concern of many other carers during the course of their day; these may be both professional and non-professional, and it is important that all are included in the pre-implant information sharing process. This serves two purposes: it ensures that the child wears the system effectively at all times and receives appropriate management, and it ensures that all concerned with the child share realistic expectations.

The team at the implant clinic

There are useful summaries elsewhere, e.g. in Fraser (1991) and Tye-Murray (1993), of the roles of each member of an implant clinic team; in paediatric implantation the main differences are the different areas of expertise required of members of the team, and the essential addition of a teacher of the deaf. The amount of work involved in paediatric implantation must not be underestimated (Goin and Parisier, 1991; Kileny, Kemink and Zimmerman-Phillips, 1991) and staff at the clinic should have prior experience in the paediatric aspects of their work to enable the establishment of close cooperation with the team at the child's home.

Team coordinator/administrator

The difficulties of multi-disciplinary work are well known (Warnock, 1986; Haggard, 1993), with misunderstandings arising among team members from different professions, but it is vital that effective coordination is achieved so that the team is seen to be providing consistent support and advice, and maintains professional credibility. At many implant centres, the coordinator is an audiological scientist; when the author's team was developed, the coordinator appointed was a teacher of the deaf, recognising from the outset the importance of establishing close liaison between a paediatric implant team and those educating the child locally (McCormick, 1991; Archbold, 1992).

With rapidly growing numbers of implanted children, often travelling long distances to the implant centres and from a wide variety of educational programmes, the problems of coordination become accordingly more complex. The coordinator's role encompasses the coordination of the role of each team member at the implant centre, as well as the interaction between the implant clinic team and those supporting the child locally. The typical tasks of a coordinator are the following:

- To respond to referrals, send out and request information.
- To manage appointments, assessments, evaluations and the database.
- To coordinate audiological, medical and rehabilitation follow-up.
- To coordinate team decisions, sharing information among team members, professional development within the team, meetings and professional visits.
- To liaise with other teams to develop 'best practice'.
- To manage the budget, order equipment and control stock.

The work of the coordinator should not be underestimated; a paediatric programme differs from an adult one in the wider range of professionals involved with each child; these professionals must feel a part of the process of implantation. This, together with the more complex assessment procedure and lengthy rehabilitation period, requires the coordinator to liaise with a large number of people for each child, both at the implant centre and at the child's home. It is important that parents and local professionals talking to a variety of team members receive consistent information and that decisions are coordinated to ensure the integrity of the programme. The coordinator should ensure that time is made for team meetings, and for sharing professional experiences, to develop a fuller understanding of the differing roles of members. In this way, implant team decisions can be made with appropriate recognition and respect for other professional viewpoints, and professional development can take place within the team. This complex coordinating role can only be achieved with a large degree of secretarial and managerial support.

Implant clinic otolaryngologists/surgeons

With young children, the surgeon has an important counselling role in addition to carrying out medical assessment before the decision to implant (Gibbin, 1992; O'Donoghue, 1992). The importance of parents' understanding of the future implications of their decision has been stressed, but parents must also make the decision to implant their child with the full knowledge of risks involved. Chapter 5 describes more fully the role of the surgeon throughout the management of the child. Although the shared responsibility of the team is stressed throughout this chapter, the surgeon carries overall clinical responsibility for the implanted child (Fraser, 1991) and there are many issues to be considered in dealing with young children. Paediatric teams find it helpful to have two surgeons, and to ensure that other members of their medical staff develop the necessary skills to provide appropriate medical cover for children. As more children are implanted who may have other disabilities, the medical assessments become more complex, and it may become necessary to liaise with other medical specialities, e.g. paediatricians, cardiologists or neurologists.

Nursing staff

The nursing staff in the hospital have a vital role to play in a paediatric implant programme; they will meet the parents and child during the assessment period, when parents may be experiencing doubts about putting their child through the tests and procedures, and concerned that their child may not be suitable for cochlear implantation. Parents may use the hospital staff to ask many of the worrying practical questions which concern them; the nursing staff must feel part of the implant programme, aware of current thinking and involved in developments within the programme. In some paediatric programmes members of the nursing staff attend team meetings to ensure full participation in the programme.

Implant clinic audiological scientists

The audiological scientists at the clinic take responsibility for full audiological assessment before implantation, including the evaluation of hearing aid use. Post-implantation, the responsibilities include the fitting and tuning of the external parts, refinements of tuning and long-term maintenance of the implant system. Further audiological investigations with and without the implant device, including sound field investigations and speech audiometry, are carried out. The scientist must discuss the external equipment, its controls and the programming process; this information must be disseminated to others in daily contact with the child. Members of the rehabilitation staff on outreach visits to home and school may be asked questions which will require further liaison with the scientist working with the child; time must be made for this liaison in the clinic. For young children with few or no communication skills, who are unable to give verbal feedback during tuning sessions, it is important that the rehabilitation team and audiological scientist work closely together so that changes in listening skills, or vocalisation, for example, are reported to the scientist. The role of the audiological scientist is developed more fully in Chapters 4 and 7.

Implant clinic medical physicist

The medical physicist works together with the audiological scientist and, in some programmes, takes responsibility for electrophysiological investigation of children. Evoked response audiometry is an essential part of the overall audiological assessment before implantation in young children, and such investigations provide an objective measure of hearing in support of behavioural tests. There is also an important role for the physicist during implant surgery and after implantation – in the development of the recording technique for the electrically evoked auditory brain-stem response (EABR) and stapedial reflexes. Electrical stimulation of the cochlea by the implant can be used to elicit the EABR. This investigation can provide valuable objective information about the functioning of the implant which can also be used to assist the later tuning-in procedure. These electrophysiological investigations are described more fully in Chapter 6.

Implant clinic technician

As large numbers of children are implanted, technical support becomes crucial. Devices break down and need repair, children need spare equipment and an efficient maintenance service must be developed. Children become dependent upon the auditory signal provided by the implant to monitor their environment as well as to access speech, and they may become very distressed if without their implant system for any length of time. This creates a great responsibility for the implant clinic to ensure reliability of technical support and its financial backing. Implant clinics must consider warranty issues, and the establishment of maintenance contracts with the supplying company. Most breakdown problems will involve returning the processor to the company, and this entails further expenditure by the team on a supply of spares.

Implant clinic teacher of the deaf

Moog and Geers (1991) expressed concern that the staff at implant clinics do not have the expertise to relate to the work being carried out in schools. In Nottingham the teachers of the deaf on the implant team take on a key worker role with the child, responsible for liaison between clinic and home/school from the initial visit to the clinic by child and family. These teachers must have wide previous experience of the different approaches and educational settings in which deaf children are placed to establish credibility in the classroom and acceptance by the child's local teacher of the deaf. The implant clinic teacher of the deaf may be required to fulfil the following various roles on visits after implantation to the child's school:

- Working with the child to demonstrate and monitor the use of the device, and ways in which it may be promoted.
- Suggesting activities which may be useful in developing listening and communication skills.
- Trouble-shooting any minor problems with the device.
- Discussing specific listening conditions and difficulties.
- Observing the child in class and individual situations.
- Helping peers as well as staff to understand ways in which they can help the child develop use of audition.
- Collecting and discussing diary entries made by staff working with the child.

These roles must be carried out sensitively; for children who have been without useful residual hearing, management styles may have been established which are counterproductive to the development of auditory competence post-implant. The object is to monitor, advise and evaluate; to ensure that the management of the child at home and at school promote the optimal use of the device.

Implant clinic speech and language therapist

The work of the speech and language therapist at the implant clinic is described in Chapter 11. As with the implant clinic teacher of the deaf, the clinic speech and language therapist visits and works with the child and the family at a local level. The speech and language therapist carries out pre-implant assessments of the child's functioning in communication skills and spoken language, with the help of parents and local professionals.

The roles outlined below are elaborated in Chapter 11:

- To describe and explain the implanted child's current communication skills.
- To demonstrate the child's readiness for speech training after implantation.
- To up-date the team speech and language therapist assessment procedure.
- To allow time for feedback on reports and for joint planning of immediate goals at all linguistic levels.
- To provide advice on appropriate materials and strategies to local professionals.

Implant clinic educational psychologist

Implant teams vary in their use of clinical as well as educational psychologists. Although cochlear implant teams have stressed that the absence of significant learning difficulties is one of the criteria, and that parental expectations and commitments should be assessed, there is very limited information about how this should be done (Laurenzi, 1993), but the expertise of an educational psychologist adds strength in this area. In the early days of implantation, implant candidates were expected to be of at least average intellectual ability, so that they could cope with the extensive pre- and postoperative testing (Aplin, 1993). It is true, particularly with the Nucleus 22 channel device, that a great deal of concentration is required from the child in lengthy tuning sessions and, until more objective methods are achieved, certain minimum levels of physical coordination and cooperation are demanded. As Laurenzi (1993) points out, however, it would be considered unethical to deny a conventional hearing aid to a child of below-average intellectual ability, and this criterion has assumed less importance.

When there is concern about a child's cognitive functioning in areas unrelated to deafness, and there is difficulty in assessing this, then the services of an educational psychologist, familiar with working with deaf children, must be obtained. After implantation, the opinion of an experienced educational psychologist may be useful in cases where a child, with lengthy access to useful audition, is not developing spoken language as expected, to determine if there is a specific learning difficulty present.

Implant clinic social worker for the deaf

The literature reports wide variability with regard to the remit of a social worker in the field of cochlear implantation. In practice, few deaf children in the UK will have access to their own social worker for the deaf, but it is important that the role is recognised by implant clinics and some use the skills of a social worker. In Nottingham, the team have a unique blend of expertise with access to a former social worker for the deaf who has herself had a cochlear implant. This provides exceptionally useful insights for parents and children, and opportunity for discussing deaf issues. Parents are encouraged to comprehend more fully that, even though their child has acquired useful audition, he or she remains deaf following implantation.

The interface between the implant clinic team and the local team

Having established the importance of the comprehensive paediatric team, including both the clinic-based team and the local professionals, the interface between them must be considered carefully. Many experienced paediatric centres recognise the importance of the interface between those based at the implant clinic and those working locally with the child. The House Ear Institute (HEI) initiated the School Contact Program in 1982, with the educators on the staff of the HEI acting in a liaison role between school and clinic (Selmi, 1985). This recognised, at an early stage in paediatric implantation, the crucial role of educators of the deaf and the value of their observations. Other implant teams in Australia, the USA, the UK and the Netherlands have developed close links with schools for the deaf, and work with teachers in their classrooms on a regular basis. The liaison offered by implant centres to local educators varies considerably, ranging from the rehabilitation being carried out mainly in the clinic with regular attendances there by parents and child, and only telephone and written contacts with the child's local professionals, to the major part of rehabilitation being in the child's own school.

In some instances, schools or classes have been established for children with cochlear implants, with teachers in charge who have specific expertise in the management of cochlear implant systems. It is arguable whether this is necessary or advisable; rehabilitation appropriate for children with cochlear implants may well be appropriate for many hearing-aided children. Implanted children do not present new problems; they are children who have useful audition following implantation, as do many hearing-aided children (Tyler, 1993b) and, as described in Chapter 8, many activities currently being used by teachers of the deaf with hearing-aided children will be suitable.

Somers (1991) recommended that implant centres in the USA should bring teachers of the deaf into programmes more actively than is currently being done. Osberger et al. (1991) describe the frustration experienced by many teachers of the deaf faced with unrealised expectations of devices and technical problems. These issues must be addressed by the implant clinic during the preparation period, so that the local teacher of the deaf, who is likely to be dealing with the daily management of the system, feels confident in handling problems and does not feel that the child has been 'dumped on them' (Beiter, Staller and Dowell, 1991). Teachers of the deaf are commonly responsible for the daily checking of hearing aid systems; although simple checks can be carried out (Chapter 7), they cannot 'listen' to the quality of the signal from the child's processor. In addition to giving input to the rehabilitation programme, the implant centre must provide information about the system's management and maintenance, and expectations of its use. This information must be provided for each new teacher the child receives; the implant clinic team bears some responsibility for ensuring that contact is maintained over time with the child's local educators, and Moog and Geers (1991) give an excellent description of the in-service training which must be provided by the implant centre for the local teachers.

The Network of Educators of Children with Cochlear Implants (NECCI) disseminates practical information for teachers of implanted children in the USA and provides a forum for discussion. In the UK, the British Association of Teachers of the Deaf, The National Aural Group and The National Deaf Children's Society encourage the sharing of expertise among teachers of the deaf, and have shown themselves willing to provide information on cochlear implantation. These are useful means by which to share general information about the management of cochlear implants, but it is still necessary for direct contact between implant centre and local professionals about the management of each specific situation: each child presents differently, and each educational setting and communication style will vary.

Educational settings

The implant clinic staff will be required to deal sensitively with a diversity of educational settings and communication philosophies, about which there is still controversy; they may also be required to work within educational settings in which they feel uncomfortable. In the UK, the communication style will range from those that are strongly oral/aural through those in which there is use of oral/aural, written and manual components (total communication) to those in which British Sign Language, with its own syntax, is considered to be the first language of the deaf child. These differing communication settings may be found in a variety of educational management settings, summarised in Table 3.1, adding to the difficulties of an implant clinic team in liaising with the local professionals.

In the first three placements in Table 3.1, the residential and day schools for the deaf and a unit without integration, there is likely to be one teacher of the deaf responsible for the child who will maintain the primary role in liaison with the implant centre. In the other settings,

Table 3.1 Range of educational management systems

Educational placement	Professional support
Residential school for the deaf	
Day School for the deaf	One teacher of
Unit for the hearing impaired	the deaf
Without integration	
With integration	
Mainstream with teacher of the deaf support/withdrawal	
Mainstream with other support/withdrawal	Range of staff
Mainstream without withdrawal	working with child
Pre-school/nursery	

where some element of mainstreaming is taking place, the implant clinic teacher of the deaf will be required to liaise with several teachers and carers who will be responsible for the child during the course of his or her day. In addition, many of these teachers and carers may have little expertise in the management of deafness, or hearing aids, let alone cochlear implants. In recent years in the UK and USA, there have been moves towards the mainstreaming of children with disabilities, i.e. the placement of these children within their local school rather than in a special school. In the UK, most profoundly deaf children are educated in integrated situations, and these offer a wide variety of support for each child, and a variety of facilities which may be acoustically unsuitable for hearing-aided, or implanted, children.

An educational outreach programme

One way in which direct contact can be developed and ongoing in-service training carried out, appropriate to the child's educational setting, is through an educational outreach programme carried out by the implant clinic teachers of the deaf and speech and language therapists. In the author's programme, this outreach programme was established at the outset, although many children live several hundred miles away. Visits are made by clinic staff to home and school at least twice before surgery and then monthly in the first year post-implantation, and every 2 months in the second and third years, as specified in Table 3.2 and in Chapter 11. In providing direct contact between implant centre and home and school, the implant professionals are able to gain some understanding of the situations in which the implant system will be functioning for most of the time, will be able to advise on the rehabilitation programme and can monitor progress with some insights into a child's individual setting. In the early days, after implantation, it will be important for the implant clinic teacher of the deaf to be able to demonstrate progress in the child's everyday settings, providing constructive feedback and support at a time when there may be little evidence of developing listening skills. In this way, parents are relieved of the burden of acting as 'go-between' from implant clinic to local educator.

The aims of this outreach programme are the following:

- To provide direct contact between implant clinic and home and school, pre- and post-implant.
- To gain insight into the child's home and educational setting.
- To ensure that the rehabilitation programme is appropriate for the child's educational setting, e.g. whatever the mode of communication.
- To ensure that the implant system is managed appropriately at home and school, so that it functions optimally at all times.

- To provide direct support and feedback for parents and local professionals.
- To monitor the development of listening skills in 'everyday' settings.

Providing direct contact with home and school is time-consuming and costly in terms of travel for the implant clinic team and the implications will be discussed later when considering staffing and long-term funding of a paediatric programme. However, by focusing rehabilitation in the child's home and school, it enables appropriate rehabilitation to be carried out throughout the child's waking hours, rather than only during clinic visits. In the author's programme, only 1% of the child's waking hours in the first year post-implantation are spent in the clinic; 99% are spent at home and school. This figure is likely to be repeated in other centres; it is essential that the implant clinic team can directly influence the use of the system during the 99% of waking hours spent away from the clinic. Working in this way can prove an effective use of the implant clinic team's time, as well as being a means of limiting the disruption to the child's family and school life, experienced when a long stay or frequent visits to the clinic are required. With more programmes in the UK working in this way, the need for the coordination of these educational outreach programmes provided by clinics to schools is becoming very evident. Staff from more than one implant centre may be working in a particular educational setting and,to maintain the support of hard-pressed educators, it is essential to ensure that visits, requests for their cooperation and advice are coordinated.

Managing a paediatric cochlear implant programme: time, staff and cost implications

Having considered the expertise necessary to carry out paediatric implant work, what are the practicalities of running such a programme? An example of the time schedule of a paediatric implant programme is given in Figure 3.3, showing progress from the initial referral through assessment, implantation, programming of the device to rehabilitation; the rest of this chapter will discuss the management of the programme through the four phases:

1. Assessment and preparation for implantation.
2. Surgery and initial fitting.
3. Rehabilitation and evaluation.
4. Maintenance.

Assessment and preparation for implantation

Other chapters will deal with candidacy issues audiologically and surgically, so a brief summary should suffice here. The following are the accepted guidelines given by Staller, Beiter and Brimacombe (1991).

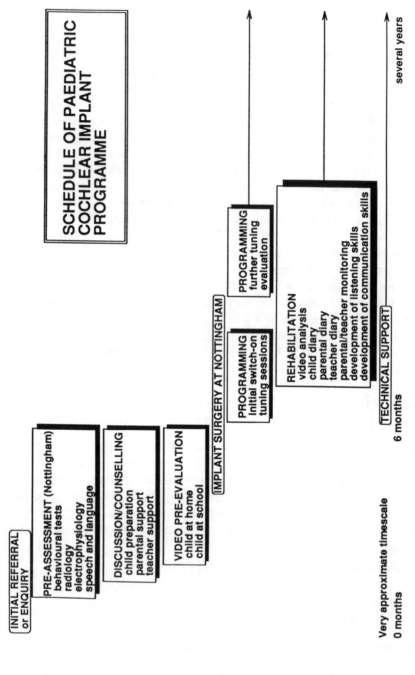

Figure 3.3 A time schedule for a paediatric cochlear implant programme

Selection criteria for children

- Bilateral profound deafness.
- Age 2–17 years.
- No radiological contraindications.
- No medical contraindications.

In addition, candidates should:

- demonstrate little or no benefit from conventional amplification;
- receive educational support which includes a strong auditory/oral component;
- be psychologically and motivationally suitable;
- have appropriate family and educational expectations and support.

Although these guidelines have been generally accepted, the audiological criteria are being challenged as experience with implants indicates the potential of these devices; a fuller discussion is given in Chapters 1 and 4.

Before the assessment phase, the coordinator at the implant clinic will have sent information to the child, the parents and the teachers, outlining the process of implantation, briefly describing a cochlear implant, the probable needs for rehabilitation and reasonable expectations from the device (Archbold, 1992; Tye-Murray, 1993). In addition, it will be important for the coordinator to obtain as much information as possible about the child, so that inappropriate cases, such as those who have very useful residual hearing, are not brought forward for assessment and parental expectations are not raised unnecessarily. This has implications for the implant centre to have available information materials that are accessible to different groups: deaf people as well as ethnic minority groups. Parents may well wish to discuss issues with the implant coordinator before the first visit; Tye-Murray (1993) summarises the most commonly asked questions, which include the practical issues of time and financial commitments required, as well as the reliability of the device and the benefits which may be expected. Parents considering implantation for their child will be particularly anxious to find out about long-term effects of the implant system, long-term support and future educational management. The coordinator may well be able to answer many questions before the assessment phase begins fully, and parents at this stage often wish to be put in contact with parents of implanted children to discuss issues with them.

Having decided to bring a child forward for assessment, the coordinator begins the arrangements for the necessary evaluations. Figure 3.4 shows the assessment protocol used by the Nottingham programme; during the assessment phase the team must carry out the following:

- audiological assessment;
- medical assessment;

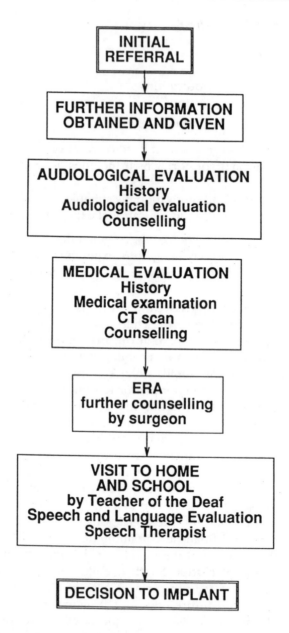

Figure 3.4 The assessment protocol used by the Nottingham Programme

- speech and language assessment;
- educational assessment;
- assessments of family expectations and commitment.

The audiological evaluation is usually carried out during the initial visit to the clinic and is described fully in Chapter 4. With the difficulties of assessing young children who have no spoken language, the audiological evaluation is the assessment at which children are most likely to be found unsuitable; this gives parents time to discuss implantation with team members before any medical intervention. It also provides a situation in which rehabilitation staff can observe the child's interaction with parents, and style of learning and communication.

If there is good reason, however, for computed tomography (CT) to take place early (e.g. following meningitis in consideration of the onset of ossification), then this procedure may be brought forward. The assessments may be deliberately spaced out at intervals so that parents have to return to the implant centre on at least three occasions; this gives parents time to reconsider their options, to formulate questions and receive answers, and to understand a little of the long-term commitment which will be expected of them. Parents have many issues to consider: the logistics of time and travel, and financial commitment, required during the rehabilitation period need careful thought. Problems that are likely to occur during the rehabilitation phase in the keeping of appointments, for example, may be brought to light during this period, as parents experience some of the difficulties which may occur in travelling to the implant centre, organising leave from work, and arranging for the needs of other members of the family to be met.

It is important during this phase that the local professionals are involved so that, should implantation not be appropriate, an informed support system is available to consider the future options for the child and to support the family in making appropriate decisions. It is also important that the family meets members of the deaf community and parents who have decided against implantation, so that all options are considered rationally. If implantation is not possible, this should not be considered as 'failure', but rather that there may be other more appropriate options for the child.

Tye-Murray (1993) lists the topics covered during counselling sessions at this stage: audiological and medical candidacy criteria, cochlear implant hardware, cost and insurance reimbursement, realistic expectations, commitment, social considerations, communication mode and educational placement. A systematic means of considering these issues and guiding decisions about candidacy has been developed by the Children's Hearing Institute, Manhattan Eye, Ear and Throat Hospital in the form of the Children's Implant Profile (CHIP) (Hellman et al., 1991). It itemises eleven factors which must be considered in assessing suitability for implantation:

1. Chronological age
2. Duration of deafness
3. Medical/radiological indications
4. Multiple handicapping conditions
5. Functional hearing

6. Speech and language abilities
7. Family support and structure
8. Family expectations
9. Educational environment
10. Availability of support services
11. Cognitive learning style.

Each factor is given a rating from a scale of 'no concern', 'mild-to-moderate concern' and 'great concern'. The whole team contributes to the completion of the CHIP, with contributions from the child's home and school professionals. The CHIP is seen as a tool in the process of decision making, not as a 'pass or fail' test of suitability. It is useful, however, in ensuring that the paediatric implant team has addressed all these issues, anticipated potential difficulties and remedied these where possible. Many difficulties, e.g. lack of available educational expertise, may not have a possible solution, although there may be alternatives available which will ameliorate the worst effects of the lack of appropriate support.

As implantation requires a long-term commitment by both the clinic team and the local team, it is vital that this assessment phase is given a priority and all concerned feel that they can contribute to the final decision. The three mains aims during this period are the following:

1. To assess the child's appropriateness for implantation.
2. To enable parents to make an informed decision regarding implantation.
3. To establish the basis for future cooperative relationships should implantation proceed (Archbold, 1992).

When the decision to implant has been taken by parents and the implant team, further and more vigorous assessments of the child's functioning are made; baselines of language and communication skills are established using standardised tests where appropriate, video analysis and observation, questionnaire and interview material. This period builds on the previous relationships already developed with child, family and local professionals, and enables full preparation of the whole team to take place before implantation.

Surgery and initial fitting

The hospital stay may be traumatic, particularly for those parents of children with hearing loss acquired through meningitis. Parents may experience re-awakened memories of the feelings of bereavement and loss experienced at the time of the acquisition of deafness. In spite of an emphasis on the development of realistic expectations, parents may still hope for a full return of hearing. As one parent commented to the author 'My head listened to you, but my heart didn't'. The responsibility for the decision to implant may weigh heavily at this time; parents bring a healthy child to hospital and choose for him or her to undergo surgery, entailing some discomfort and risk. Their feelings may be difficult to share with professionals; parents have found it helpful that the author's team carry out operations on two children at the same time, so that they can be mutually supportive. The ward staff have a crucial role to play, and they need to understand the nature of the whole process and the comparatively brief, but vital, role of surgery in the programme. This can be a useful period for developing a further understanding of family dynamics which may later influence the rehabilitation programme.

The surgery itself and management are described in Chapter 5; although the surgeon's role is the critical one at this time, the team as a whole must be available to support the family. This support is particularly important if postoperative complications develop.

After discharge, a few days after the operation, the children in the Nottingham programme are visited at home by the implant clinic teacher of the deaf, and prepared, with their families, for the next stage – the initial tuning of the device. They are able to familiarise themselves with the equipment and its controls, decide how they will wear the processor, see photos of other children, share books about it and prepare for listening experiences in a realistic way. Older children may be prepared more specifically for the activities that tuning in the device will require of them; highly structured preparation for the tasks ahead, however, is not necessary and the child may well not understand the concepts involved in tuning the device without the experience of sound stimulation.

The initial tuning session is often called 'Switch-on'; this is rather a misnomer, but is taken to mean the time at which the external parts of the device are fitted – microphone, transmitter and processor – and is described fully in Chapter 7. This takes place some 4 weeks after surgery, and with young children the initial tuning period is generally 3 days. As Osberger (1986) clarifies, there are three main aims at this time:

1. To set the device.
2. To assess the responses of the child.
3. To enable parents and professionals to plan the programme for the development of listening skills.

The rehabilitation staff and audiological scientists liaise closely; it is mutually useful to share the child's responses in the clinic and outside world. Eisenberg (1985) comments that many parents are concerned primarily with the perception of environmental sounds for safety reasons; this is an area in which immediate responses are often observed and early rehabilitation consists of 'listening walks' and having fun with sound. Play with sound makers and musical instruments develops the child's confidence and pleasure in using the device before carrying out more structured listening tasks – both linguistic and non-linguistic. The final day of the initial visit may involve the child's local teacher of the deaf, speech and language therapist and audiologist so that they can learn how to manage the system and promote its use at home. With the child wearing the device at comfortable listening levels, we can move into the rehabilitation phase.

Rehabilitation and evaluation

With the benefits of implantation only being seen in the long term, the importance of the entire team and the preparation phase is now 'tested' as the team begins to function for a period of several years. The rehabilitation phase involves implant clinic scientists, teachers, and speech and language therapists working with the family, and local professionals to ensure optimum use of the device and the attachment of meaning to sound by the child. Appropriate rehabilitation activities are described in Chapter 8; the implant clinic team must ensure that:

- Parents and teachers are able to maintain the device appropriately.
- Spares are available at all times, and everyone knows how to trouble-shoot the device.
- The child is in optimum conditions to use the new sense of audition, bearing in mind the educational setting and style of communication.

Although the author's team has emphasised the importance of the implant clinic team's visits to home and school, the child and family will need to visit the implant centre at regular intervals. During these visits (usually 8 days in the first year in the Nottingham programme – see Table 3.2) the child will see the surgeon, audiological scientist, speech and language therapist and teacher of the deaf at the clinic, and will have:

- a medical check;
- further tuning of the device;
- monitoring of the system;
- evaluation of listening skills;
- evaluation of spoken language skills;
- discussions of progress so far and guidelines for further progress.

This rehabilitation phase should last for at least 3 years, and others have recommended at least 5 years; concerns by educators express the need for continued liaison as children change teachers or schools (Moog and Geers, 1991). It is the responsibility of the implant centre to ensure that this long-term commitment and liaison is possible, ensuring continuity in use of the device for children.

Maintenance

As implantation may result in the altering of communication style, educational management, career options and how the child later perceives him- or herself (Tyler, 1993b), the statement that implantation involves a commitment for life (Goin and Parisier, 1991) is not far from the truth. The maintenance phase must last for the life of the child, with, at the very least, regular maintenance of the system, the availability of spares, repairs and a trouble-shooting service. With growing recognition of some of the technical problems encountered with equipment (Tyler and Kelsay, 1990), this maintenance period is vital.

After the 3-year postoperative rehabilitation programme, the Nottingham team provides at least an annual clinic visit, together with a maintenance contract for all hardware problems, a contact service for local professionals and medical cover. The author's team has found it useful to provide the child with an identity bracelet from a medical security firm which makes details of the child's implant and any medical conditions available anywhere in the world in the case of an emergency.

Staff and cost implications of a paediatric cochlear implant programme

There has been little published work to itemise the staffing and cost implications of a paediatric implant programme, although its time-consuming and costly nature has been recognised (Goin and Parisier, 1991; Kileny, Kemink and Zimmerman-Phillips, 1991), and Tye-Murray (1993) discusses the cost issues experienced by implant candidates in the USA. Having established the life-long support needed by implanted children, and the increasing awareness of complexities of maintaining implanted devices, it is essential that paediatric implant programmes look to their long-term funding and staffing. It is equally important that, in order to cost their programme accurately, all elements of the service are included and that purchasers of the programme, whether health authorities, insurance companies or individuals, are able to know what they are buying and the length of the financial commitment.

Table 3.2 shows one example of information material available for purchasers: this was sent, with a brochure, to all health care purchasers in the UK by the Nottingham programme. It itemises costs for

Table 3.2 Programme contents and costs 1994–1995

	Year 1	Years 2 and 3	Year 4 onward
Assessments			
Audiological	*		
Medical	*		
Speech/language	*		
Educational	*		
ERA	*		
CT	*		
Preparation			
Child	*		
Family	*		
Local professionals	*		
Implant and surgery	*		
Tuning of processor	*(8)	*(3)	*(1)
Device support			
Emergency repairs	*	*	*
Immediate replacements	*	*	*
Reasonable maintenance costs	*	*	*
Regular medical checks	*(6)	*(3)	*(1)
Rehabilitation			
Monitoring of device	*(8)	*(3)	*(1)
Monitoring of progress	*(8)	*(3)	*(1)
Home visits	*(12)	*(6)	
School visits	*(12)	*(6)	
Support group	*	*	*
Cost	£27 000	£4000 p.a.	£2000 p.a.

*The Nottingham Paediatric Cochlear Implant Programme, based at both the General and University Hospitals, was established in 1989.

Number in parentheses indicate *minimum* numbers of visits. Tuning and rehabilitation visits involve a full day. Additional provision will be included as required.

The full programme of payments above allows for the purchase of a *new speech processor* after 6 years, as recommended by the manufacturer.

Nottingham has an international reputation for research. Patients benefit from spin-off from the various research projects, all of which are separately funded by additional grants.

Our level of support has ensured that all our implanted children are 100% full-time users of the device, allowing maximum benefits from implantation.

1994–1995, and the service provided. These costs allow for the level of support described in this chapter, including rehabilitation and full maintenance of the device, and replacement processors. To produce accurate information of this kind, the financial and time implications of the programme need to be considered in some detail. A database has been developed at the author's programme in collaboration with the Medical Research Council's Institute of Hearing Research, which enables staffing, time and equipment cost inputs to be monitored, as well as maintaining biographical data and outcome measures on children. The time spent by staff during visits by the child to the implant centre, or by implant clinic staff to the child, are itemised under the following categories:

- audiological evaluation;
- fitting and maintaining hardware;
- assessment;
- medical checks;
- rehabilitation;
- family counselling;
- liaison with other professionals;
- travel to home and school.

The time inputs given to each child during the period 1989–1993 by the Nottingham Paediatric Programme have been measured; graphs of total time commitment by staff per implanted child (excluding travel) are given for a 4-year period post-implantation in Figure 3.5. The first year is the most labour intensive, but, in contrast to an adult

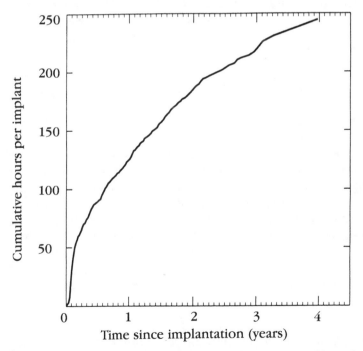

Figure 3.5 The total time commitment by staff/implanted child (excluding travel) during a 4-year period post-implantation: the experience of the Nottingham team 1989–1993

Average Number of Staff Activity hours per Child

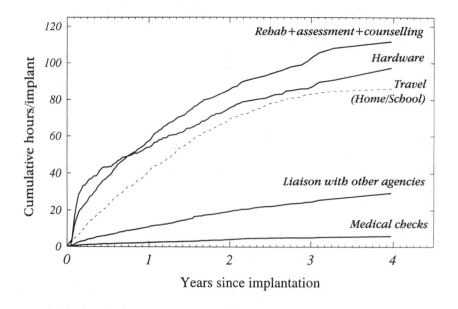

Figure 3.6 The time commitment by staff/implanted child broken down by categories: fitting and maintaining hardware, travel, assessment, rehabilitation, family counselling, liaising with other professionals and medical checks. The experience of the Nottingham team, 1989–1993

programme, in years two and three following implantation, children continue to require considerable support from the implant clinic. Figure 3.6 reveals the amount of time spent in fitting and maintaining hardware, travelling to home and school by the implant clinic staff, assessment, rehabilitation, family counselling, liaising with other professionals and medical checks. The time spent in family counselling and liaising with other professionals enables the implant clinic team to influence the management of the implant system directly when the child is at home and school, so that full benefit is developed throughout the child's waking hours, not only when visiting the clinic. It may well be that, in time, the amount of time spent per implanted child will be reduced, as more local professionals gain direct experience of working with implanted children. This is being monitored, but already appears to be occurring.

The use of accessible outcome measures for health care purchasers

Although recognising the need for rigorous outcome measures in children, conventional measures of speech perception and production do

not enable a health service purchaser or financial adviser to comprehend what an implant may offer a deaf child. Implant programmes
must provide evidence of the efficacy of implantation in an accessible
form to purchasers to obtain long-term funding. Table 3.3 shows an
example of one way in which the functional benefit from implantation
may be represented. Listening performance has been classified according to the following scale:

- No awareness of environmental sounds.
- Awareness of environmental sounds.
- Response to speech sounds, e.g. 'go'.
- Identification of environmental sounds.
- Discrimination of some speech sounds without lipreading.
- Understanding common phrases without lipreading.
- Understanding conversation without lipreading.
- Use of telephone with known speaker.

The table also classifies performance of the first 40 children implanted
in Nottingham. Before implantation, only two children were able to
respond to the loudest sounds with conventional aids. Apart from a
child with specific language difficulties, all the implanted children who
had their devices for 3 years were able to understand conversation
without lipreading and to monitor their environment via audition; two
(one-third) were able to use the telephone. This performance classification is undergoing further refinement and development, but has
proved useful in presenting information about the benefit obtained by
children following implantation to health care purchasers.

Conclusion

Other chapters in this book clarify the specific demands made on the
cochlear implant team by the implantation of young deaf children. At
the time of writing, guidelines are being established in the UK for the
minimum standards required for paediatric implantation. They were
drawn up by Barry McCormick, as principal author, in consultation
with implant professionals representing all implant programmes in the
UK. They are supported by the British Cochlear Implant Group and the
National Deaf Children's Society and include the following:

- Multi-disciplinary teams with relevant paediatric experience.
- Specialist centres, implanting at least 10 children per annum.
- Established educational networks.
- Long-term commitment and funding.
- Dedicated staff for the paediatric teams.

Taking the child as the focus of the programme, Figure 3.7 illustrates
the triangle of support necessary to ensure the long-term effectiveness

Table 3.3 Performance in young children before and after cochlear implantation

Before implant (n=40)	Category of performance	0 months (n=40) (at initial tuning)	6 months (n=32)	12 months (n=25)	24 months (n=15)	36 months (n=6)
	Use of telephone with known speaker		1		1	2
	Understanding of conversation without lipreading		1	1	6	3
	Understanding of common phrases without lipreading				5	
	Discrimination of some speech sounds without lipreading	6	18	23	3	1
	Identification of environmental sounds		7	1		
	Response to speech sounds (e.g. 'go')	17	5			
2	Awareness of environmental sounds	17				
30	No awareness of environmental sounds					

Nottingham Paediatric Cochlear Implant Programme (August 1993): number of children achieving each category.

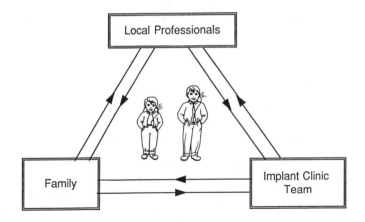

Figure 3.7 The triangle of support necessary for the child

of the device, with the local team of professionals, implant clinic team and family working together with the child. Paediatric implantation involves a long-term financial and time commitment (Goin and Parisier, 1991), which is only being recognised with experience, and a paediatric programme must be based on sound management to ensure its future viability for all implanted children. Given the indications of long-term benefit which are emerging from implant teams throughout the world, this is a field which deserves planned expansion.

Acknowledgements

The author gratefully acknowledges the work of Dr David Marshall of the MRC Institute of Hearing Research, Nottingham in developing the database which is used in managing the Nottingham programme, and for colleagues and Professor Mary Joe Osberger of Indiana University School of Medicine for comments on this chapter.

References

Aplin, D.Y. (1993) Psychological assessment of multi-channel cochlear implant patients. *Journal of Laryngology and Otology* **107**, 298–304.

Archbold, S. (1992) The development of a paediatric cochlear implant programme: A case study. *British Journal of the Association of Teachers of the Deaf* **16** (1), 17–26.

Bamford, J. and Saunders, E. (1991). *Hearing Impairment, Auditory Perception and Language Disability*, 2nd edn. London: Whurr.

Beiter, A.L., Staller, S.J. and Dowell, R.C. (1991). Evaluation and device programming in children. *Ear and Hearing* **12** (4), 25S–33S.

Boothroyd, A. (1989). Hearing aids, cochlear implants and profoundly deaf children. In E. Owens and D.K. Kessler (eds), *Cochlear implants in Young Deaf Children*, pp. 81–100. Boston: Little, Brown and Co.

Cayton, H. (1991). Problems and issues in developing a cochlear implant programme for children. *Journal of Medical Engineering and Technology* 15 (2), 49–52.

Conrad, R., (1979). *The Deaf School Child*. London: Harper and Row.

Downs, M.P. (1986). Psychological issues surrounding children receiving cochlear implants. In D.J. Mecklenburg (ed.) *Cochlear Implants in Children: Seminars in Hearing*, pp. 383–406. New York: Thième Medical.

Eisenberg, L.S. (1985). Perceptual abilities with the cochlear implant; Implications for aural rehabilitation. *Ear and Hearing* 6, 60S–69S.

Evans, J.W. (1989). Thoughts on the psychological implications of cochlear implantation in children. In E. Owens and D.K. Kessler (eds), *Cochlear Implants in Young Deaf Children*, pp. 307–314. Boston: Little, Brown and Co.

Fraser, G. (1991). The cochlear implant team. In H. Cooper (ed.), *Cochlear Implants: A Practical Guide*, pp. 84–91. London: Whurr.

Geers, A.E. and Moog, J.S. (1991). Evaluating the benefits of cochlear implants in an educational setting. *American Journal of Otology* 12, 116–125.

Gibbin, K.P. (1992). Paediatric cochlear implantation. *Archives of Disease in Childhood* 65, 669–671.

Goin, D.W. and Parisier, S.C. (1991). Implementing a cochlear implant team in private practice or academic setting. *American Journal of Otology* 12, 213–217.

Haggard, M. (1993). *Research in the Development of Effective Services for Hearing Impaired People*. Fifth H.M. Queen Elizabeth the Queen Mother Fellowship, The Nuffield Provincial Hospital Trust, London.

Hellman, S.A., Chute, P.M., Kretschmer, R.E., Nevins, M.E., Parisier. S.C. and Thurston, L.C. (1991). The development of a children's implant profile. *American Annals of the Deaf* 136 (2), 77–81.

Kessler, D.K. and Owens, E. (1989). Conclusions: current considerations and future directions. In D.K. Kessler and E. Owens (eds), *Cochlear Implants in Young Deaf Children*, pp. 315–330. Boston: Little, Brown and Co.

Kileny, P.R., Kemink, J.L. and Zimmerman-Phillips, S. (1991). Cochlear implants in children. *American Journal of Otology* 12 (Suppl. 2), 144–146.

Kirk, K.I. and Hill-Brown, C. (1985). Speech and language results in children with a cochlear implant. *Ear and Hearing* 6 (Suppl. 3), 36S–47S.

Laurenzi, C. (1993). The bionic ear and the mythology of paediatric implants. *British Journal of Audiology* 27, 1–5.

Lea, A.R. (1991). *Cochlear Implants: Australian Institute of Health*. Health Care Technology Services, 6, AGPS, Canberra.

Luterman, D. (1987). *Deafness in the Family*. Boston: Little, Brown and Co.

McCormick, B. (1991). Paediatric cochlear implantation in the UK – a delayed journey along a well marked route. *British Journal of Audiology* 25, 145–149.

Mecklenburg, D.J., Demorest, M.E, and Staller, S.J. (1991). Scope and design of the clinical trial of the Nucleus multichannel cochlear implants in children. *Ear and Hearing* 12 (Suppl. 4), 10S–14S.

Moog, J.S. and Geers, A.E. (1991). Educational management of children with cochlear implants. *American Annals of the Deaf* 136 (2), 69–70.

O'Donoghue, G.M. (1992). Cochlear implants in children. *Journal of the Royal Society of Medicine* 85, 655–657.

Osberger, M.J. (1986). Auditory skill development in children with cochlear implants. In D.J. Mecklenburg (ed.), *Cochlear Implants in Children: Seminars in Hearing*, pp. 423–432. New York: Thième Medical.

Osberger, M.J. (1990). Audiological rehabilitation with cochlear implants and tactile aids. *ASHA* **32**, 38–43.

Osberger, M.J., Dettman, S.J., Daniel, K., Moog, J.S., Siebert, R., Stone, P. and Jorgenson, S. (1991). Rehabilitation and education issues with implanted children: perspectives from a panel of clinicians and educators. *American Journal of Otology* **12**, 205–212.

Power, D.J. and Hyde, M.B. (1992). The cochlear implant and the deaf community. *Medical Journal of Australia* **157**, 421–422.

Quigley, S.P. and Kretschmer, R.E. (1984). *Language and Deafness*. London: Croom Helm.

Quittner, A.L., Thompson Steck, J. and Rouiller, R.L. (1991). Cochlear implants in children: A study of parental stress and adjustment. *American Journal of Otology* **12**, 95–104.

Selmi, A. (1985). Monitoring and evaluating the educational effect of the cochlear implant. *Ear and Hearing* **6** (3), 52S–59S.

Somers, M.N. (1991). Effects of cochlear implants in children: implications for rehabilitation. In H. Cooper (ed.), *Cochlear Implants: A Practical Guide*, pp. 322–345. London: Whurr.

Staller, S.J., Beiter, A.L. and Brimacombe, J.A. (1991). Children and multichannel cochlear implants. In H. Cooper (ed.), *Cochlear Implants: A Practical Guide*, pp. 283–321. London: Whurr.

Tye-Murray, N. (1993). Aural rehabilitation and patient management. In R.S. Tyler (ed.), *Cochlear Implants: Audiological Foundations*, pp. 87–144. London: Whurr; San Diego: Singular.

Tyler, R S (1993a). Cochlear implants and the deaf culture. *American Journal of Audiology* March, 26–32.

Tyler, R.S. (1993b). Speech perception by children. In R.S. Tyler (ed.), *Cochlear Implants: Audiological Foundations*, pp. 191–256. London: Whurr; San Diego: Singular.

Tyler, R.S. and Kelsay, D. (1990). Advantages and disadvantages reported by some of the better cochlear implant patients. *American Journal of Otology* **11**, 282–289.

Warnock, M. (1986). Children with special needs in ordinary schools: integration revisited. In A. Cohen and L. Cohen (eds), *Special Educational Needs in the Ordinary School*. London: Harper & Row.

Webster, A. (1986). *Deafness, Development and Literacy*. London: Methuen.

Wood, D.J., Wood, H.A. Griffiths, A.J. and Howarth, C.I. (1986). *Teaching and Talking with Deaf Children*. London: John Wiley.

Chapter 4
Assessing audiological suitability of implants for children below the age of 5 years

BARRY McCORMICK

Introduction

Assessment of candidacy for cochlear implantation requires a full and detailed clinical audiological evaluation, which may extend from 1 to 4 hours in duration. The resulting clinical findings must then be considered in the light of the child's performance at home and in any available educational setting. The methods and principles detailed in Chapters 8, 9, 10 and 11 of this book will be essential for this purpose.

This chapter concentrates on the evaluation of clinical findings to determine whether the implant might be suitable for the child and not whether the child might be suitable for the implant. The child-centred approach must not be overlooked when viewing the range of findings from the test procedures. The child and his or her family have needs, and the audiological evaluation helps to determine whether the implant system of choice might play some part in helping to satisfy one of those needs.

It is probable that assessments from an expertly staffed and well-equipped department will unearth basic audiological needs in some children which have not been met by their local service. The conveyance of tips and exchange of ideas among the services might benefit children for whom the implant route is not considered to be appropriate at that stage, but for whom alternative techniques are indicated. The implant audiological assessment must be very reliable and use state-of-the-art techniques. It can be anticipated that advice on improved hearing aid and earmould provision might be all that is required in some cases. This has certainly been the experience in a significant number of children who have been referred to the Nottingham programme. Many families have commented that their children have never been tested thoroughly before or that the child has never cooperated to the same degree. Some parents are surprised that their child can or will sustain a good response pattern, and it is often very rewarding for the family to witness the child's abilities during the implant assessment sessions.

A very common finding has been that basic hearing levels have been obtained previously but no testing had been undertaken under hearing-aided conditions. Without such evaluation, it is impossible to know whether the child might gain additional help from a cochlear implant. Requests for previous aided threshold measurements sometimes meet with the response that facilities for undertaking such measurements are not available locally. The facilities required in terms of equipment are minimal and it is normally expertise that is lacking.

Another problem encountered when trying to assess audiological suitability for implantation is the presence of middle-ear effusion. The existence of a conductive hearing loss of unknown, even if only of very slight, degree will prevent the obtaining of true hearing-aided responses which represent typical rather than temporarily reduced hearing levels. It can be very frustrating for families to travel a long distance to an implant centre, only to discover that the assessment cannot be performed because of the presence of middle-ear effusion. Steps need to be taken to avoid such abortive journeys by arranging for medical and/or surgical assessment and treatment in the weeks before the audiological assessment.

The assessment sequence

The approach adopted within the Nottingham programme is that the paediatric audiological assessment should precede and not follow the medical, radiological and electrophysiological testing (with the exception of the check for and treatment of any conductive hearing disorder). The reasoning for this reflects some of the findings reported above and the fact that it is imperative that optimum hearing aid use has been secured for some considerable time, thus permitting the benefits, or lack of benefit, of the systems to be determined. It would be wasteful of the surgeon's time for detailed discussion to take place between parents and surgeon about the surgery and aftercare if basic audiological testing can confirm that the implant route is not appropriate for the child. The limitations of acoustic amplification can be assessed by the paediatric audiologist in consultation with the parents, the education team, and the speech and language therapist.

An exception to this test sequence might be made in the case of children deafened by meningitis for whom the risks of new fibrous growth (ossification) within the cochlea might prevent the later insertion of a multichannel intracochlear implant. In these cases early radiology might be indicated to assess the patency of the cochlear ducts.

In the absence of ossification, caution must be exercised in cases of deafness following meningitis because of the possibility of recovery of hearing even after total deafness. Such a case has been documented by McCormick et al. (1993) and the lesson is that in the absence of ossification there should be a period of watchful waiting, probably extending to at least 6 months, during which time the effectiveness of hearing aid use can be determined. A minimum of 6 months of hearing aid use is desirable for all children regardless of the cause of deafness (Beiter, Staller and Dowell, 1991), and most children will have a much longer trial than this.

Liaison with the child's local audiological assessment service is essential and any previous audiological findings should be made available. For the actual appointment, the child should be equipped with good earmoulds and these, together with the ear, nose and throat investigations to exclude middle-ear problems, should be subjected to consideration during the few weeks immediately before the appointment at the implant centre.

The investigations

A 90-minute session is recommended for the first appointment to allow sufficient time to obtain a comprehensive audiological profile. A settling-in period should be allowed with the child playing with attractive toys while a history is taken and the hearing aids are given a full technical performance check.

Hearing aid condition and technical performance

The state and physical condition of the hearing aid may indicate the extent of its use. Suspicions of lack of use might be raised if the aids show no signs of wear and tear, in spite of having been issued for some considerable time with no replacement. It is vital to know, and be reassured, that hearing aid use had been given a fair trial over many months to give credence to the assessment of benefit or lack of benefit. Most parents accept this requirement, but sometimes the trial might, unfortunately, be foreshortened by the parents if no overt signs of benefit are apparent in the first few months or if the child rejects the instruments.

The condition of the earmould and tubing should be inspected to see if the tubing is loose or hard and discoloured with age, and to check that the mould is not blocked with wax or debris. It may be necessary to renew the tubing and/or clean the mould in an ultrasonic cleaner. If body-worn hearing aids are used, the presence and condition of the receiver washers should be checked with replacements being fitted if necessary.

Hearing aid electroacoustic performance should be checked using a well-calibrated test station, plotting the gain, frequency response, harmonic distortion and, if possible, intermodulation distortion according to standard procedure (IEC, 1983 abc or ANSI, 1987). It is also desirable to measure the performance of the aid set on the user's normal volume, tone, maximum output and other internal settings, with an input corresponding to a typical speech level of 60 dB.

Assessing hearing threshold

The technique for measuring hearing thresholds will vary according to the age of the child. The basic techniques will be distraction testing for babies below 2 years of age, pre-conditioning for performance testing from 2 to 2½ years and full performance testing and conventional audiometry beyond 2½ years. Visual reinforcement methods can be used throughout this period, but it is normally most successful from 18 months onwards.

The distraction test

This test has been described in detail elsewhere (McCormick, 1993) and space does not permit the coverage to be repeated here. The technique can be used with babies from 5 months of age, and sometimes below this age if the child's head and spine are suitably supported. Head-turn responses are elicited to a variety of frequency-specific sounds presented outside the baby's peripheral vision, following a sequence of attention capture and phasing to ensure that the baby is in a suitable state to respond. Intense noises with strong vibrotactile components can be used, although these will inevitably not be frequency specific in nature. A particular merit of the distraction technique is that the baby's responsiveness, or lack of responsiveness, to the modalities of sound, touch and vision can be assessed simultaneously, or in quick sequence, to check on the state of awareness and attention. If a child turns quickly to a touch on the ear from behind or to an object brought into peripheral vision, but does not turn to sound, this is indicative of a hearing loss. Lack of response to all three modalities will indicate something about the child's attention state, but not necessarily the presence or extent of a hearing problem.

Localising responses under hearing-aided conditions can be elicited with post-aural hearing aids, but not necessarily with body-worn instruments (see later discussion on aided thresholds). Visual reinforcement methods might be more appropriate for body-worn hearing aid assessment.

The distraction techniques can be used beyond the age of 12–18 months, but it becomes more problematic and the child's increasing social awareness can render the test invalid if he or she consistently searches for the person who is presenting the noise stimuli. The technique of visual reinforcement audiometry may be more satisfactory.

Visual reinforcement audiometry

A detailed account of this technique is given by Bamford and McSporran (1993) and coverage of the finer points of detail will not be given here. Basically, stimulus sounds are presented through a speaker arrangement and the child's orientation response is rewarded with some visual display (e.g. the lighting of eyes on a toy animal). In the early part of the test, the child is conditioned to turn towards the speaker by associating the sound stimulus with the light reward (classical conditioning), and later the light reward is given only if the child correctly turns to the speaker when a sound stimulus is present (operant or instrumental conditioning). With this technique the sound can be presented from the front or from either side, and the light reward can be presented adjacent to or remote from the speaker. Some advocates of the technique do not make claims about the testing of each ear individually when speakers, rather than headphones, are used. The technique can, therefore, be used to obtain aided responses through body-worn hearing aids because the child is conditioned to look towards the light rather than to locate the source of sound.

Normally the child's responses are observed through a one-way observation window from a control room which houses the sound delivery and light reward controls. One of the problems with the method is that it is not possible to present very high stimulus levels, which would be tolerable for the parent or for another worker in the room unless headphones were used. Such equipment might prove to be disturbing to some children. A variation of the techniques has been described by Bamford and McSporran (1993) in which insert earphones can be used and high stimulus levels can be presented through the child's own earmoulds.

The requirement for high stimulus level presentation can be met in the distraction test technique by holding the signal generator speaker immediately adjacent to the child's ear or hearing aid microphone while remaining outside the field of vision. By these means, it is quite possible to present stimuli in excess of 100 dB to the child without distressing others in the room.

It will be appreciated that visual reinforcement audiometry (VRA) and distraction techniques both have advantages and limitations, and information gained from each should be exploited to the full in an attempt to obtain the maximum number of aided and unaided responses from the very young child. The significance of the responses obtained and their values will be discussed later in this chapter.

The performance test and pure-tone audiometry

From the age of 2 years, some children, and from the age of 2½ years most children, can be conditioned to wait for a sound stimulus (or light or vibrotactile stimulus) and to respond to this in a simple play activity. This 'performance' technique marks a significant transition in test technique, with the child now actively cooperating in a task which provides pre-conditioning for pure-tone audiometry at a time when headphones or a bone vibrator might not be tolerated.

The testing can be undertaken in a sound field setting with or without hearing aids. For a child with a very limited concentration span, who is on the borderline for conditioning to the task, it might be wise to undertake the 'aided' investigation first and establish the conditioning with a stimulus containing a strong vibrotactile component. Once the response pattern is established, acoustic stimuli should be used as soon as possible; if there is no response to these, the vibrotactile stimuli should be re-introduced to check consistency. The use of light stimuli might also be useful and the child can be trained to respond when a small light illuminates. The significance of any lack of response to acoustic stimuli in the hearing-aided and -unaided conditions can be determined by checking the consistency, or lack, of response to the three modalities.

A useful technique for the vibrotactile element in the test is to hold the bone vibrator on the child's hand and to introduce a 250 Hz tone at 40 dB. The vibrations from this stimulus can be felt very easily and a few guided responses should soon establish the conditioning. The vibrator can then be introduced to the mastoid, perhaps by holding it gently against the head to extend the 'game'. Some children will reject the headband at first and the equipment should, therefore, be introduced cautiously to maintain the child's cooperation.

Conditioning with light or vibrotactile stimuli will be essential for most children for whom the suitability of cochlear implantation is being assessed and typical vibrotactile levels have been given by Boothroyd and Cawkwell (1970). These are summarised in Table 4.1. Many children evaluated within the Nottingham programme have demonstrated vibrotactile bone-conduction levels of 50 dB HL at 500 Hz and it may be that very young children have a greater sensitivity to such stimulation. There is considerable individual variation and, although it is not possible to give definitive values, the pattern of vibrotactile response is quite clear and there is normally a discrete lack of responsiveness to such stimuli above 1 kHz (certainly within the range of most audiometer outputs). This marked cut-off reassures the tester that the conditioning is reliable and response pattern consistent.

Suitable play materials are shown in Figure 4.1. Anything with a facility for repetition of a simple play activity will be useful and the

Table 4.1 Typical vibrotactile threshold levels

Conduction	Threshold levels (dB HL) at frequency of		
	250 Hz	*500 Hz*	*1000 Hz*
Air	80–110	100–120	120–130
Bone	20–40	55–70	80–85

After Boothroyd and Cawkwell (1970).

success of the test will depend to a significant extent on the novelty of the task and the ingenuity of the tester to be adaptable and flexible with the materials. Frequent changes of games may be required with, for example, a wooden man being nudged off the table into a box rather than placed in a boat, after the child's interest in the boat has been exhausted. It is vital that the child should not receive any visual cue other than during the conditioning phase or when the light stimulus is used deliberately. The period between stimulus presentations should be varied in an unpredictable manner to ensure that the child is not simply forming a set response pattern. Delays in stimulus presentation from 1 to 10 seconds should be included in a random sequence.

A few guided responses from the tester will be required to establish the conditioning and as a general rule if the child does not show any restraint, but just responds impulsively, after 20 guided/demonstration responses this verifies that the child does not have a sufficient level of maturity for the task. If conditioning does not appear to be successful it will, of course, be necessary to ensure that the child is perceiving a sufficient signal, either visual, auditory or vibratory.

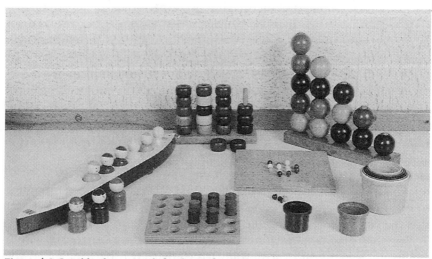

Figure 4.1 Suitable play materials for the performance test

Ideally headphones or a calibrated sound-field system should be used but if very high output levels are required and the child will not accept headphones it will be necessary to hold the sound stimulus directly adjacent to the child's hearing aid microphone, or the child's ear, and this can be achieved either by gently holding the earphone of the audiometer over the child's ear, or by holding a hand-held signal generator in close proximity to the ear or hearing aid microphone. The level can then be measured with the generator held at the same distance from the microphone of the sound level meter.

Hearing thresholds under hearing-aided and -unaided conditions should be determined using the standard Hughson and Westlake ascending technique (described by Carhart and Jerger, 1959), whenever possible, although with the very young child it might be necessary to use fairly gross ascending steps of 10 dB rather than 5 dB to bracket the area of the threshold if it is clear that the child's cooperation will be maintained for only a short interval. If a good response pattern can be maintained it is desirable to undertake the aided response threshold recordings using 2-dB or even 1-dB incremental steps after initially establishing the threshold in 5-dB ascending steps. The thresholds can be recorded in decibels hearing level (dB HL) (with pure tones presented through headphones) or decibels (A) (dB(A)) or decibels sound pressure level (dB SPL) if sound-field warble tone recordings are made. Conversion factors will be needed if the sound field values are to be plotted in dB HL on a conventional audiogram form. Such conversion factors have been given by Lutman and McCormick (1987) and these are reproduced in Table 4.2. In practice it is more convenient, and more consistently accurate, to record the responses in the scales in which they are measured, and it is acceptable to plot these on an audiogram form if a clear note is made to the effect that the responses are to warble-tone stimuli and they are in dB(A) or dB SPL and not dB HL.

Table 4.2 Conversion factors from dB(A) to HL equivalent

Frequency (Hz)	Conversion (dB(A) to dB SPL)	Minimal audible field (binaural) (dB SPL from ISO-226)	True conversion values (dB(A) to dB HL equivalent)
250	+9	+12	−3
500	+3	+6	−3
1 000	0	+4	−4
2 000	−1	+1	−2
4 000	−1	−4	+3
8 000	+1	+15	−14
10 000	+3	+16	−13

From Lutman and McCormick (1987).

Interpreting the significance of the hearing thresholds

An illustration of a combined aided and unaided response pattern is given in Figure 4.2. In this example there is considerable improvement in the thresholds under the condition of hearing aid use. The anticipated gain from the hearing aid amplification can be checked approximately from the 2 cm³ coupler measurements or with improved accuracy using 2 cm³ to real ear conversion factors for babies or children. With some children it might be possible to record insertion gain measurements with a probe microphone in the ear canal and to use computer-assisted hearing aid selection procedures (for example Seewald, Moss and Spiro, 1985).

Such techniques will not be discussed further in the context of this chapter and the interested reader is referred to Seewald, Moss and Spiro (1985) and Green (1993) for details of the procedures. Such selection procedures are not so applicable for the very profound hearing loss category and most children brought forward for cochlear implant assessment will be wearing powerful hearing aids and will not show the expected acoustical gain from the systems. A typical response pattern for such a case is given in Figure 4.3 and it can be seen that this differs markedly from the efficient hearing aid user's result in Figure

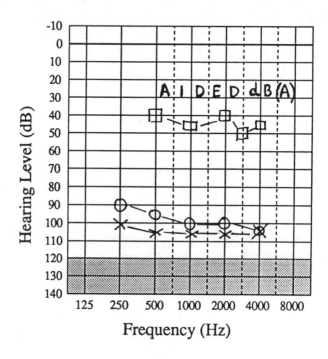

Figure 4.2 An example of an audiogram showing aided and unaided thresholds for an efficient hearing aid user. The aided responses are to warble tone stimuli and they are measured in dB(A)

4.2. These two illustrations represent extreme examples and there is, of course, a range of possibilities between these two extremes.

Figure 4.4 shows approximate areas of aided responses which correspond to efficient and effective hearing aid use. These areas indicate trends and have been derived from retrospective analysis of such measures, obtained by the author over a decade from children attending his department. The early aided responses have been compared with the actual performance levels of the children up to 10 years later, when only minor changes have been made to the aided response pattern following the provision of updated hearing aids over that period. The author concluded from this retrospective surveillance exercise that children with aided responses of less than 60 dB across the frequency range 500–4000 Hz were likely to be efficient and effective hearing aid users, and those with aided responses in excess of 60 dB were not likely to benefit significantly. Examples of actual case findings for efficient users are given for cases A, B and C in Figures 4.5, 4.6 and 4.7, and the corresponding scores for these three cases in a closed set speech discrimination test without lipreading are:

Case A   93% at 45 dB(A)
Case B   >90% at 70 dB(A)
Case C   70% at 60 dB(A)

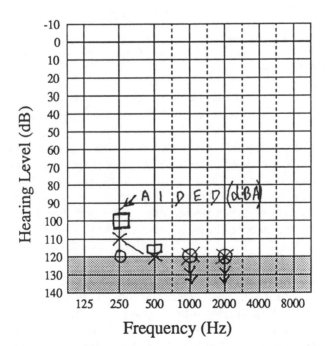

Figure 4.3 A typical aided and unaided response pattern for a profoundly/totally deaf child who shows no benefit from amplification. The aided responses are to warble tone stimuli and they are measured in dB(A)

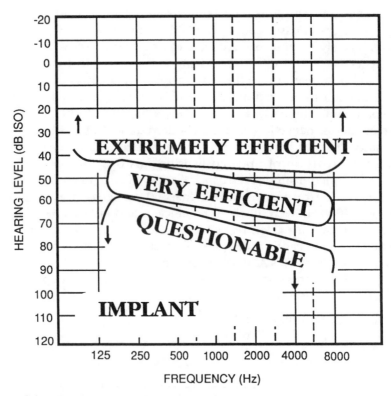

Figure 4.4 Aided threshold prediction of hearing aid benefit. Aided threshold response patterns obtained from the files of children attending the Children's Hearing Assessment Centre, Nottingham

In contrast the typical aided and unaided findings for a non-effective hearing aid user (case D) are given in Figure 4.8; this child is unable to score above chance in a closed set speech discrimination task without lipreading and even with lipreading he obtains a very low score only just above the chance level. This finding is not surprising when the typical areas of concentration and distribution of sounds in conventional speech are plotted on an audiogram (Figure 4.9) on which his responses are superimposed. It can be seen that his aided thresholds fall outside this area. It is accepted that a person with a hearing loss in excess of 60 dB will not develop spoken language skills without amplification. If amplification does not reach the area of the speech spectrum, it can be anticipated that there will be major problems.

It was the author's surveillance of the files of children who were not progressing well with hearing aids (5 years ago) that led to the search for an alternative form of support, and to the audiological justification for the formation of the Paediatric Cochlear Implant Programme in Nottingham. The above, rather simplistic, aided threshold guide developed at that time has still proved to be of value in assessing cochlear

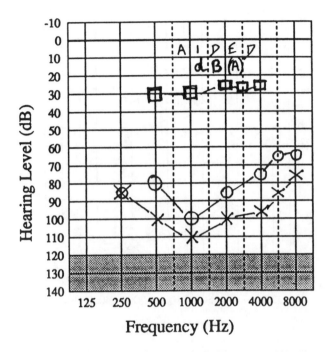

Figure 4.5 Aided and unaided audiogram for an efficient hearing aid user (case A)

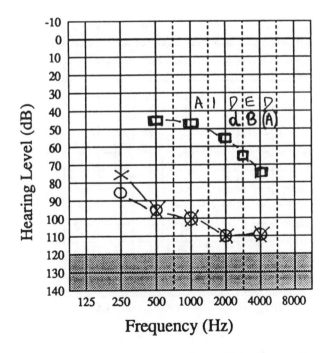

Figure 4.6 Aided and unaided response pattern for an efficient hearing aid user (case B)

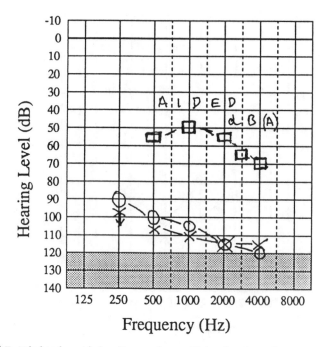

Figure 4.7 Aided and unaided audiogram for an efficient hearing aid user (case C)

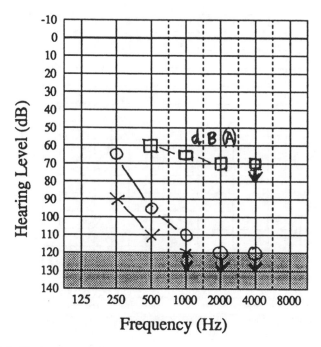

Figure 4.8 Aided and unaided audiogram for an non-efficient hearing aid user (case D)

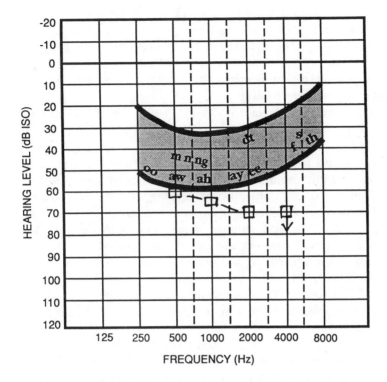

Figure 4.9 Distribution of the sounds of speech at conversational (60 dB) level plotted on an audiogram (shaded area) with the aided response pattern for case D superimposed

implant candidacy. More refined approaches to hearing aid user categorisation have been developed by other workers including Osberger et al. (1991) and Boothroyd (1993), and it is interesting to note that, although the categorisations have been derived by different (albeit related) means, the final conclusions are very similar.

Osberger et al. (1991) adopt an approach which uses unaided hearing threshold categories for profoundly deaf hearing aid users. These are based on the average unaided thresholds at 500 Hz, 1 kHz and 2 kHz and three categories are described:

1. Bronze – unaided thresholds averaging >110 dB HL.
2. Silver – unaided thresholds averaging 101–110 dB HL.
3. Gold – unaided thresholds averaging 90–100 dB HL.

The bronze users are potential candidates for cochlear implant assessment and they fall within the present author's questionable/implant area, taking into account the realistic hearing aid gain achievable across the frequency range 500–2000 Hz. The silver users might be potential candidates, in that they can be expected to fall within or just outside the present writer's questionable area for efficiency of hearing aid use.

The final decision about their suitability will depend to a large degree upon their performance after prolonged hearing aid use. The gold hearing aid users should fall into the present writer's very efficient hearing aid user category, and as such will not be potential candidates for cochlear implantation unless their performance with hearing aids after years of use is very poor.

Further data from Miyamoto et al. (1993) on children who have used implants for 3 years or more indicate that the implant users often out-perform silver hearing aid users, and they approached the level of gold hearing aid users. It was concluded that silver hearing aid users might derive more benefit from a multichannel cochlear implant than from continued use of conventional hearing aids. It is also conceivable that, with more experience, the implant users might surpass the gold hearing aid users in performance. Given that gold hearing aid users should, with good hearing aid provision, fall within the writer's 'extremely efficient' hearing aid users' category, implant teams could face a real dilemma because of the significant increase in the numbers who might be suitable for evaluation within their programme. Work is under way to investigate this matter further at both Nottingham and Indianapolis.

The above, rather optimistic and ambitious, future application for cochlear implants is not shared by Boothroyd (1993) who states that it is difficult to justify implantation unless the hearing loss is 110 dB or more (i.e. within the present writer's 'questionable' category), but he qualifies this by stating that any decisions should involve more extensive assessment of auditory capacity and performance. In an earlier paper (Boothroyd, Geers and Moog, 1991), it was stated that if a person failed to demonstrate auditory capacity in spite of good pure-tone thresholds, proper amplification and adequate listening experience, then the possibility of cochlear implant benefit should be given more weight. Boothroyd, Geers and Moog (1991) chose to classify auditory capacity of severely and profoundly deaf children operationally as the ability to perceive, in varying context, significant contrasts among acoustic speech patterns when wearing hearing aids. It is interesting to relate the typical findings from their categorisations with the audiometric levels in Table 4.3. These categorisations provide an additional link between the unaided thresholds and probable speech discrimination performance, although it must be noted that there can be considerable variation within the 90–110 dB group and this has been demonstrated by Erber and Alencwicz (1976). It is, therefore, of particular importance to have evidence of effectiveness and efficiency of hearing aid use, based on informed observations of a very young child's performance at home and in any educational setting. Sensitive measures, such as those presented in Chapters 8–11 in this book, are required.

When the Nottingham programme was first launched, the only

Table 4.3 Classification of auditory capacity of severely and profoundly deaf children

Hearing loss (dB HL)	Contrasts perceived
>110	Only those cued by relatively slow amplitude variations (e.g. vowel height, vowel duration, syllable pattern)
90–110	Above, together with relatively robust spectral patterns (e.g. pitch rise and fall, vowel place) and those cued by rapid variations of amplitude over time (e.g. initial consonant, voicing, consonant manner)
<90	Above, plus subtle spectral patterns and rapid variations of spectrum over time (e.g. place of articulation of consonants)

After Boothroyd, Geers and Moog (1991).

children who could be considered for assessment were those who demonstrated vibrotactile response patterns with no evidence of any response to acoustic signals (McCormick, 1991). With further experience of the application of the technique, and of its advantages, and with increasing general acceptance of cochlear implantation, the criteria for eligibility were relaxed to include children with aided responses of 80 dB or more. More recently, children with 60/70 dB aided responses have been considered if they also satisfy the requirement of lack of progress with hearing aids. It is likely that in the future children with low-frequency aided responses in the region of 40–50 dB and high frequency responses in the region of 60–70 dB will be considered if there is clear evidence of lack of progress with hearing aids after prolonged trials. The justifications for inclusion of such children will be on the basis of the high-frequency advantage offered by the implant, and the documented progress of children with similar histories who have shown rapid progress after implantation.

The foregoing discussion has assumed that the thresholds obtained are stable with no superimposed conductive hearing loss. Despite the fact that a recent otological assessment is a prerequisite before the audiological assessment appointment it cannot be assumed that middle-ear fluid is not present on the day and it is essential to test for this. Tympanometry is the standard clinical procedure for obtaining information about middle-ear transmission function. A diagram of the middle-ear structures was given in Chapter 2 (Figure 2.1).

Tympanometry

When to test

Although it is desirable to undertake tympanometry recordings at the start of the session, it is often wise to postpone these to towards the end if it is suspected that the child might reject the equipment. The child's cooperation should be retained at all cost, and introducing equipment that might be rejected early in the long test session could spoil all chances of obtaining and sustaining essential response patterns. It is inevitable that the application of this cautious regime will sometimes mean that considerable efforts will be expended to obtain thresholds, which cannot then be interpreted reliably if tympanometry indicates the presence of a conductive hearing loss.

The procedure

Tympanometry or middle-ear impedance (the reciprocal of admittance) measurement involves reflecting a sound wave off the ear drum (tympanic membrane) and measuring the intensity of the reflected sound. This gives an indication of the sound energy that is absorbed by the middle-ear structures. In the static state, this can be done with a single measurement of 'reflectivity', but it is much more useful and informative to undertake a dynamic measurement using the following procedure.

The air pressure in the external canal is inflated, and measured, by means of a pump and manometer arrangement, so that it is slightly above atmospheric pressure. This induces a pressure loading on the tympanic membrane and hence more sound will be reflected. The pressure is then reduced until it is slightly below atmospheric pressure, thus causing the tympanic membrane to be tense but this time in the opposite direction. Between the two extremes, there will be a point of balance when the pressure on both sides of the tympanic membrane is equal. This will occur at atmospheric pressure if the middle ear is well ventilated by the eustachian tube. At this point the tympanic membrane will be flaccid and the incident sound wave will be absorbed easily. The measure of the variation of the reflected sound in the ear canal with the change in air pressure will enable the tympanogram to be plotted, and this will have various configurations according to the state of the middle ear. If there is fluid present, there will be restricted movement of the system and a stiffening of the tympanic membrane causing the trace to be flat (Figure 4.10). If the middle-ear pressure is normal there will be a peak in the curve corresponding to atmospheric pressure (Figure 4.11). If the middle-ear pressure is reduced there will be a reduced peak at a negative pressure relative to the atmospheric pressure (Figure 4.12). There are, of course, other possibilities but the above represent the main traces of interest and others will need more expert interpretation by the paediatric audiologist in consultation with the otologist.

The normal trace will provide reassurance that there is no significant conductive hearing loss in all but a very rare number of cases, and

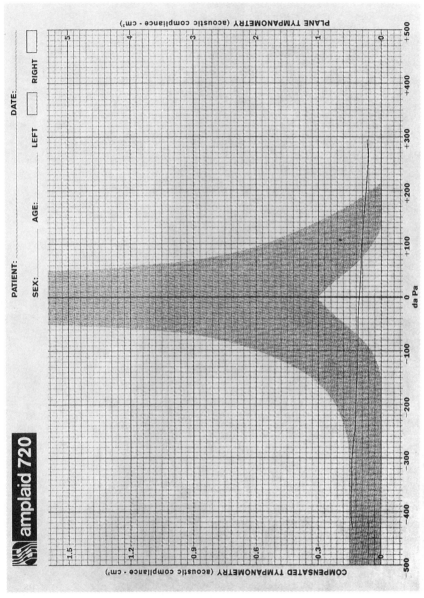

Figure 4.10 Tympanogram showing a flat trace

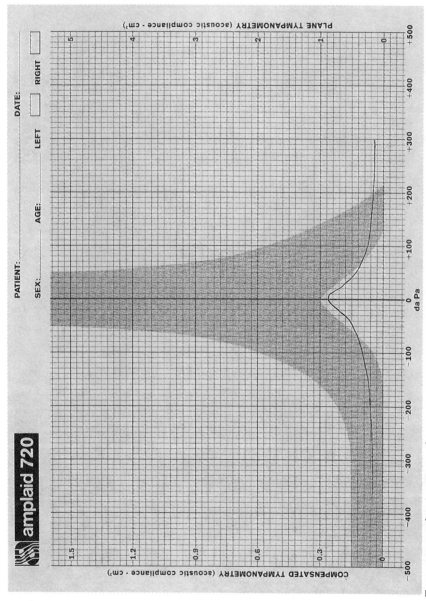

Figure 4.11 Tympanogram showing a normal trace

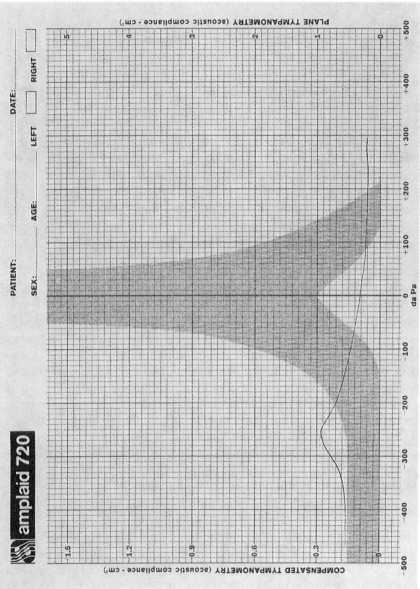

Figure 4.12 Tympanogram showing a negative middle-ear pressure and reduced compliance

the technique can be extended to include the measurement of stapedial reflex activity. Stimulation of one ear with an intense signal (e.g.
pure-tone or narrow band noise in excess of 70 dB) will trigger the
contraction of the stapedial muscle in both ears, in subjects with normal hearing, and those with reduced hearing and abnormal loudness
recruitment. This muscle contraction changes the impedance of the
middle-ear structures and tenses the tympanic membrane. Stimuli up
to 100–110 dB can be used to determine the presence or absence of
the reflex. The presence of the reflex demonstrates the intact nature of
the auditory tract up to the level of the brain stem and hence the technique offers a fairly objective additional check on the child's responsiveness or lack of responsiveness to acoustic stimuli. Although it is
unlikely that the reflex will be present in any child referred for cochlear
implant evaluation, the test should still be used routinely in all cases
demonstrating normal middle-ear mobility. Further coverage of tympanometry and its wider applications is given by Brooks (1993).

Otoacoustic emission measurements (cochlear echo)

This is another test for which a negative finding can be expected. The
recording of otoacoustic emissions (OAEs) provides a means by which
the possibility of a retrocochlear lesion could be indicated (i.e. a lesion
beyond the cochlea). Clearly, the cochlear implant would not provide
useful stimulation if the mechanism linking the cochlea to the higher
auditory tract is not functioning.

The phenomenon of otoacoustic emissions, or 'cochlear echo', was
first reported by Kemp (1978) and a full review of its application is
given by Cope and Lutman (1993). If a very sensitive microphone is
placed in the external ear canal and click stimuli are presented, it is
possible, with appropriate circuitry, to record the presence of acoustic
emissions which originate from within the healthy cochlea. These emissions are believed to arise from the active biomechanics of the cochlear
sensory mechanism at the pre-neural level. If they are present, the indication is that any hearing loss is probably retrocochlear in origin. This
would then be a contraindication to cochlear implantation. A case
study demonstrating the value of the technique for indicating lesions
has been reported by Lutman et al. (1989). The emissions are record-
able only if there is no conductive hearing loss and it is important,
therefore, to obtain the middle-ear impedance recordings first.

Patuzzi (1993) has provided a framework for classifying cochlear
and retrocochlear lesions, and he stresses that we need to divide these
into those that affect the mechanical activity within the cochlea, and
presumably the otoacoustic emission, and those that do not.

Otoacoustic emissions are early sensations to the motor component
of any lesion (outer hair cell mechanico-electrical and electro-mechanical

transduction) and not to the sensory process (including inner hair cell mechano-electrical transduction). As there are very few cases of pure sensory losses in the experimental literature and no clear-cut cases in the human clinical literature, the fact that otoacoustic emissions might not detect the sensory aspect of the mixed (sensory and motor) loss is not considered to be a problem in using otoacoustic emission tests.

Recording the otoacoustic emissions should be attempted during the initial assessment session, although if the child is too active, or rejects the equipment, it might be necessary to defer this test until the occasion when the electrophysiological tests are carried out under sedation (see Chapter 6). The electrophysiological tests may indicate further evidence of any retrocochlear disorder.

The absence of otoacoustic emission activity will offer some degree of reassurance that the lesion is within the cochlea but this test, and none of the tests discussed so far, can give any indication of whether there is a sufficient degree of neuron survival for an implant to provide stimulation. A technique of stimulating the middle-ear promontory or round window with an electrical stimulus from a needle electrode has been used with adults and older children who can report subjective impressions of any stimulation they perceive, but this is inappropriate for the very young. The true prognostic value of this technique has yet to be determined. The reader is referred to Chapter 6 for further details of promontory stimulation.

Speech discrimination tests

An aspect of assessment which might be inaccessible to the very young, particularly candidates for cochlear implant assessment, is that of speech discrimination testing. Most cases are brought forward because they are not demonstrating any progress with hearing aids and they show no ability to understand or perceive words or sentences through their hearing aids. Nevertheless attempts should be made to assess visual, auditory and audiovisual speech discrimination performance to establish a baseline measure from which to judge future progress.

The author's Toy Discrimination Test (McCormick, 1977) was developed for use with very young children with a mental age from 2 years, and it has found widespread application in audiology clinics. The test material (Figure 4.13) can be presented with or without lipreading or gesture and, because it uses some of the first words known to children, in its reduced form, it can be used for children as young as 18 months. The details of its application will not be presented here for they have been given full and recent coverage elsewhere (McCormick, 1993), but basically the test consists of a series of seven paired toy items known to the typical 2-year-old child. Each pair has been chosen to have the maximum possible acoustical overlap within the constraints of a child's

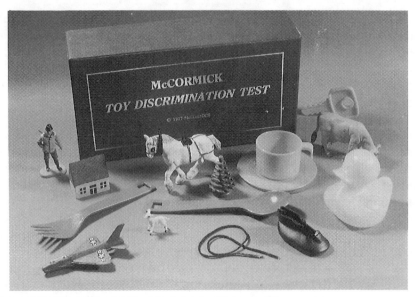

Figure 4.13 The McCormick Toy Discrimination Test material

vocabulary at this age. The paired items known to the child are displayed and the child is required to point to each item on request. The listening level at which the child obtains an 80% score (four correct responses from five requests) is recorded and represents the reference level from which future changes and performance can be assessed. If a child responds to the items with gesture and lipreading, but does not respond in the pure auditory mode or does not show any improvement in response when the auditory signal is presented through hearing aids, then this clearly demonstrates the limitation of hearing aid use for speech discrimination purposes.

It is most unlikely that any child who demonstrates an ability to make use of auditory information to improve performance in this test would be considered for further evaluation within a cochlear implant programme. Most children can, however, perform this test without lipreading within 2 or 3 years of receiving a cochlear implant and the baseline measure of a zero performance before implantation assumes relevance and significance. A further extension of the technique that has proved to be of enormous value within the Nottingham programme after implantation is the IHR/McCormick Automated Toy Discrimination Test (Ousey et al., 1989; Palmer, Sheppard and Marshall, 1991). In this version of the test (Figure 4.14) the words are recorded on microchip memory and they are presented through a speaker arrangement. The scores are logged automatically within an adaptive response procedure, all under microprocessor control. All the tester has to do is keep the child's attention on the task and press a button to score each response. This automated version of the test provides a very precise score with good control over parameters and variables which are less well defined in the live version of the test. It is not, of course, possible to include lipreading or audiovisual assessment in the auto- mated version and in the context of the pre-implant assessment the live version of the test is still needed.

The automated version has proved to be of particular value for assessing children after implantation and, again, the zero score obtained for all cases before implantation can be contrasted to the excellent levels of performance after a few years' experience with the implant. Most of the children in the Nottingham Programme have been able to perform the automated test within 3 years of receiving their implants with the criterion 71% discrimination score being achieved at listening levels of 40–60 dB(A). Work is in progress to exploit the potentials of this test further including the use of the speech-in-noise option.

Given that no child for whom the cochlear implant is considered appropriate will be able to obtain a score in the live or automated ver- sion of the Toy Discrimination Test when tested in the auditory-only mode, it is essential that the evaluation techniques specified in Chapters 8–11 are used to establish the base level performance in audi- tory detection and auditory discrimination tasks.

Conclusion

The audiological assessment fulfils a crucial function within a paedi- atric cochlear implant programme, and it must include an assessment

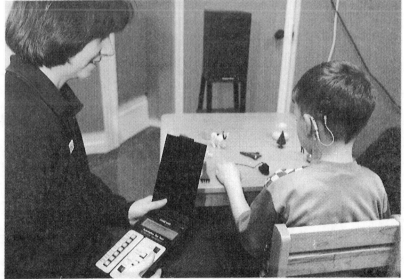

Figure 4.14 The Institute of Hearing Research (IHR)/McCormick Automated Toy Discrimina- tion Test

of the state and effectiveness of hearing aids, aided and unaided hearing thresholds, middle-ear impedance measurements, otoacoustic emission measurements and speech audiometry. At any stage in this test sequence, it may become apparent that the child's needs are not for cochlear implantation but for some alternative support or provision. If the implant route is not the one best favoured, it will be necessary to allow time to counsel the family and to explain the significance of the findings in relation to the child's needs.

No family should leave the clinic feeling abandoned by the implant programme because the child does not fit within the implant criteria. It is inevitable that some parents will have focused their minds on an implant and will consider it the solution to the child's communication difficulties. Such feelings and aspirations are natural and the implant team must handle these with empathy and point out that there are other viable and positive alternatives. Other families will show a sense of relief that the implant may not be appropriate and feel that they have served the child well by exploring all possibilities. It is essential that the paediatric audiologist should involve the teachers of the deaf, the surgeon, the speech and language therapist, and other members of the team in making final decisions, particularly when children are marginal candidates.

As experience widens and the advantages of cochlear implantation and its benefits become more apparent, it is inevitable that more children will be implanted from the marginal and questionable hearing aid user category. Implant teams face a real challenge during this period of rapid evolution of the technique.

References

ANSI (1987). *American National Standards: Specification of Hearing Aid Characteristics:* ANSI S3.22. New York: American National Standard Institute.

Bamford, J. and McSporran, E. (1993). Visual reinforcement audiometry. In B. McCormick (ed.), *Paediatric Audiology 0–5 years*, 2nd edn, pp. 124–154. London: Whurr.

Beiter, A.L., Staller, S.J. and Dowell, R.C. (1991). Evaluation and device programming in children. *Ear and Hearing* 12 (Suppl. 4), 25S–33S.

Boothroyd, A. (1993). Profound deafness. In R.S. Tyler (ed.), *Cochlear Implants: Audiological Foundations*, London: Whurr.

Boothroyd, A. and Cawkwell, S. (1970). Vibrotactile thresholds in pure tone audiometry. *Acta Oto-Laryngologica* 69, 381–387.

Boothroyd, A., Geers, A.E., Moog, J.S. (1991). Practical implications of cochlear implants in children. *Ear and Hearing* 12 (Suppl. 4), 81S–89S.

Brooks, D.N. (1993). Acoustic measurement of auditory function. In B. McCormick (ed.), *Paediatric Audiology 0–5 years*, 2nd edn, pp. 291–311. London: Whurr.

Carhart, R. and Jerger, J.F. (1959). Preferred method for clinical determination of pure tone thresholds. *Journal of Speech and Hearing Disorders* 24, 330–345.

Cope, Y. and Lutman, M.E. (1993). Otoacoustic emissions. In B. McCormick (ed.),

Paediatric Audiology 0–5 years, 2nd edn, pp. 250–290. London: Whurr.

Erber, N.P. and Alencewicz, C.M. (1976). Audiological evaluation of deaf children. *Journal of Speech and Hearing Disorders* **41**, 256–267.

Green, R. (1993). Hearing aid selection and evaluation for pre-school children. In B. McCormick (ed.), *Paediatric Audiology 0–5 years*, 2nd edn, pp. 355–377. London: Whurr.

IEC (1983a). *Measurement of Electroacoustic Characteristics*. IEC Publication 118-0. Geneva: International Electroacoustical Commission.

IEC (1983b). *Hearing Aids With Automatic Gain Control Circuits*. IEC Publication 118-2. Geneva: International Electroacoustical Commission.

IEC (1983c). *Measurement of Performance Characteristics of Hearing Aids for Quality Inspection for Delivery Purposes*. IEC Publication 118-7. Geneva: International Electroacoustical Commission.

Kemp, D.T. (1978). Stimulated acoustic emissions from within the human auditory system. *Journal of the Acoustical Society of America* **64**, 1386–1391.

Lutman, M.E. and McCormick, B. (1987). Converting free-field A-weighted sound levels to hearing levels. *Journal of the British Association of Teachers of the Deaf* **11**, 127–129.

Lutman, M.E., Mason, S.M., Sheppard, S. and Gibbin, K.P. (1989). Differential diagnostic potential of otoacoustic emissions: A case study. *Audiology* **28**, 205–210.

McCormick, B. (1977). The Toy Discrimination Test: an aid for screening the hearing of children above the mental age of two years. *Public Health (London)* **91**, 67–73.

McCormick, B. (1991). Cochlear Implantation in the U.K.: A delayed journey on a well marked route. *British Journal of Audiology* **25**, 145–149.

McCormick, B. (1993). Behavioural hearing tests 6 months–3;6 years. In B. McCormick (ed.), *Paediatric Audiology 0–5 years*, 2nd edn, pp. 102–123. London: Whurr.

McCormick, B., Gibbin, K.P., Lutman, M.E. and O'Donoghue, G.M. (1993). Late partial recovery from meningitic deafness after cochlear implantation: A case study. *American Journal of Otology* **14** (6), 1–3.

Miyamoto, R.T., Osberger, M.J., Todd, S.L., Robbins, A.M., Karasek, A., Dettman, D., Justice, N. and Johnson, D. (1993). *Speech perception skills of children with multichannel cochlear implants*. Paper presented to the Third International Cochlear Implant Conference, Innsbruck, Austria, April 1993, in press.

Osberger, M.J., Robbins, A.M., Miyamoto, R.T., Berry, S.W., Myers, W.A., Kessler, K.K. and Pope, M.L. (1991). Speech perception abilities of children with cochlear implants, tactile aids or hearing aids. *American Journal of Otology* **12** (Suppl.), 105–115.

Ousey, J., Sheppard, S., Twomey, T. and Palmer, A.R. (1989). The IHR/McCormick Automated Toy Discrimination Test: description and initial education. *British Journal of Audiology* **23**, 245–249.

Palmer, A.R., Sheppard, S. and Marshall, D.M. (1991). Prediction of hearing thresholds in children using an automated toy discrimination test. *British Journal of Audiology* **25**, 351–356.

Patuzzi, R. (1993). Otoacoustic emission and the categorisation of cochlear and retrocochlear lesions. *British Journal of Audiology* **27**, 91–95.

Seewald, R.C., Ross, M. and Spiro, M.K. (1985). Selecting amplification characteristics for young hearing-impaired children. *Ear and Hearing* **6**, 48–53.

Chapter 5
Medical aspects of paediatric cochlear implantation

KEVIN P. GIBBIN and GERARD M. O'DONOGHUE

Paediatric cochlear implantation requires input from many health care professionals (Gibbin, 1992; O'Donoghue, 1992). However, it clearly needs to be recognised that surgical involvement includes not only the actual implantation but also the preoperative assessment, counselling of parents and others, as well as the postoperative care of the child (and his or her parents!) and the management of any medical problems that may subsequently arise. It is essential that the surgeon is intimately involved at all stages of the implant process. Although cochlear implantation is now a well-established procedure in children, it is still – and in the view held at Nottingham, correctly – carried out in only a limited number of centres; it requires surgical expertise of the highest order and, as is apparent from the other chapters in this book, requires the integration of many different skills, all of which need to be readily available on one site to ensure the success of what is a major event in the child's life. The ultimate responsibility for the decision to operate and overall responsibility for the care of the child lie with the surgeon who carries out the operation, that decision being guided by colleagues in other disciplines. The surgeon 'carries the can'!

Preoperative assessment

The medical assessment of a child for cochlear implantation covers a number of important areas before a decision to implant can be taken. These may be summarised as follows:

1. The degree of deafness.
2. Aetiology of the deafness – the diagnosis of the cause.
3. Otological assessment – including diagnosis and treatment of other factors contributing to the deafness.
4. Radiological assessment.

5. General medical evaluation including an assessment of such factors as general developmental progress and general medical conditions which may affect the outcome.
6. Overall interpretation of the audiological and other data resulting from the assessment process.

Most children will have been referred to the surgeon at the implant centre by an otologist or audiological physician in the child's home town and much will already be known about the child's medical background, including the probable diagnosis of the cause of the deafness, possible middle-ear pathology and other related medical problems. Similarly, the referring doctor will have already obtained an assessment of the child's hearing loss and will have given the child a trial of appropriate hearing aids. In spite of all this, it is normal practice to complete a full reassessment, both audiologically and medically, including a full otological evaluation, at the implant centre.

It is the practice within the Nottingham Paediatric Cochlear Implant Programme for a child referred for possible cochlear implantation to be assessed audiologically as a first step. At this point some children will be gauged as unsuitable because of hearing levels above those considered appropriate for implantation or because the child has not been given an adequate trial of an appropriate hearing aid. However, once assessed as being within the audiological criteria, the child will be seen by the otologist in the team for medical and otological assessment.

Otolaryngological assessment

At this stage the surgeon will carry out a full ENT clinical examination and also assess the child's general medical condition. Otological examination will be looking particularly for evidence of active middle-ear disease; this may include a history and other evidence of recurrent acute otitis media and of course otitis media with effusion (OME). More rarely there will be underlying chronic suppurative otitis media which may need medical or surgical attention.

The role of OME in the management of severe sensorineural deafness is well understood – even a minor additional hearing loss resulting from the presence of a conductive component in a child with a severe or profound sensorineural deafness may be enough to prevent that child from gaining benefit from even the most powerful of hearing aids. Clearly therefore any underlying OME will need to be treated to be able to assess the purely sensorineural component of the deafness; it is our practice to advise myringotomy and insertion of grommets in these cases. Following this a further audiological assessment will be required. If a decision to implant is taken, then before the implantation surgery is carried out, the grommets will need to be removed if they have not extruded naturally.

Children who present with a history of recurrent acute otitis media will need additional evaluation; any factor predisposing to recurrent infections will need to be sought and attention paid to treating it. It is in this context that adenoidal enlargement and a history of possible adenoiditis or other upper respiratory tract pathology may need consideration; if there is a history of mouth breathing, snoring, night-time cough or frequent upper respiratory infections, and there is evidence of adenoidal hypertrophy, then adenoidectomy may need to be carried out. In some children with a history of persistent upper respiratory tract infection, other measures may also be needed including maxillary sinus washout and possibly a long course of a suitable broad-spectrum antibiotic. All these measures are intended to help reduce the risk of recurrent otitis media.

Other middle-ear disease will need to be carefully assessed; a perforated ear drum is a contraindication to cochlear implantation in that ear, although it may still be possible and appropriate to consider implanting the other ear, bearing in mind the strictures already referred to in the context of an additional conductive component. Reconstructive middle-ear surgery may therefore be required to repair a perforated tympanic membrane to achieve a more normal ear and to eliminate any conductive loss resulting from the perforation. More rarely, there may be damage to the ossicular chain and this may need tympanoplastic surgery; this particular problem has not been encountered in the Nottingham programme.

Attico-antral disease will similarly require treatment on *a priori* grounds; its presence will delay implantation in the diseased ear until it can be certain that all residual disease has been eliminated. Alternatively, it will force the decision that the other ear will have to be the one implanted. One such case has been encountered in the Nottingham programme.

Diagnosis of the cause of the deafness is all important because a misdiagnosis can potentially result in a child being inappropriately implanted, for example, if there is a retrocochlear cause for the deafness and there is no, or only limited, eighth nerve function; an alternative example is denial of an operation when benefit would have been gained by the child from such a procedure. Careful history taking is therefore essential and liaison may be needed with various other specialists including, in particular, clinical geneticists and paediatricians. The surgeon will be assisted in ensuring that the loss is cochlear rather than retrocochlear by carrying out brain-stem evoked response audiometry. Similarly, if otoacoustic emissions are elicited this would again be evidence of a neural deafness and a contraindication to cochlear implantation.

Although the medical history will reveal the cause of the hearing loss in most cases, physical examination may demonstrate abnormalities to explain the deafness – for example, evidence of one of the many deafness syndromes.

In many instances the diagnosis will be clear, for example, after meningitis, and the issue then becomes one of suitability for implantation on other grounds. Meningitis presents its own special problems with the possible development of new bone growth within the lumen of the cochlea – labyrinthitis ossificans or cochlear osteoneogenesis. This occurs in approximately one-third of cases of profound hearing loss resulting from meningitis; although it usually involves only the first few millimetres of the basal turn of the cochlea, it may be sufficient to obstruct the lumen completely so preventing use of an intracochlear device. The radiological examination will provide essential information.

Radiological assessment

Radiological examination of the temporal bones is a fundamental part of the preoperative assessment of a child for cochlear implantation; a number of points need to be examined including the delineation of anatomical structure and the diagnosis of disease. Accurate appraisal of the cochlear coils is vital before the insertion of an intracochlear device and it has been suggested that implantation of the Ineraid device requires better preoperative radiology than the Nucleus device because its design requires a sufficiently patent scala tympani to allow insertion of the electrodes.

Thin section high-resolution computed tomography (HRCT) is the most widely employed method of imaging the inner ear and neural pathways at present, although magnetic resonance imaging (MRI) may have a role to play in demonstrating the presence of fluid within the cochlea. In children both CT scanning and MRI at best require sedation to ensure that the child remains sufficiently still to obtain satisfactory pictures; in very young children a general anaesthetic is needed.

Ultra-high resolution CT scanning produces contiguous 1-mm sections to delineate the anatomy of the inner ear and adjacent structures, the sections being taken in both the coronal and axial planes giving increased definition and detail to this area. The Nottingham experience (Bath et al., 1994) supports results from elsewhere with an 87% accuracy in predicting absence of intralabyrinthine ossification in cases of deafness resulting from meningitis. Figure 5.1 demonstrates a normal CT scan. However, in 15% of cases the degree of ossification is underestimated; another 12% of cases demonstrated fibrosis within the scala tympani which was not detected by radiology. Figure 5.2 shows ossification of the cochlea.

It is possible that MRI may provide further information; this technique allows the visualisation of the presence or absence of fluid within the cochlear turns and would therefore appear to lend itself to the

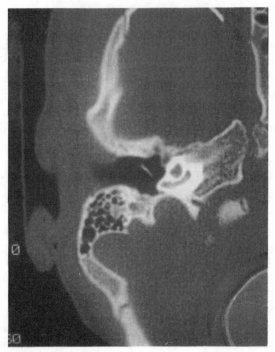

Figure 5.1 Normal high-resolution CT (HRCT) scan. (Courtesy of Drs Holland and Jaspan)

assessment of children deafened by meningitis and congenitally deaf children. It has been reported that, using a combination of these two methods of imaging, there were no surprises as to the status of the cochlea during surgery (Laszig et al., 1988).

In addition to imaging the cochlea, adjacent structures need to be evaluated including the internal auditory canal and eighth nerve pathways, the mastoid air cell system and the thickness of the squamous temporal bone where the implant package will be located.

In cases of deafness caused by meningitis, debate exists about when children should be assessed radiologically in the light of possible cochlear ossification (and subsequently how soon such children should be implanted). It is not known how soon after meningitis ossification occurs, one suggestion being that it behaves much like fracture callus after a bony fracture – possibly a matter of weeks later. This would then support early imaging in these cases with a view to possible early implantation – the debate continues.

The other major group of children likely to receive cochlear implants is the congenitally deaf group. Satisfactory radiology in these cases is essential to be aware of congenital inner ear malformations such as Mondini's where there might be a high risk of abnormal cerebrospinal fluid (CSF) communication with the inner ear fluids and

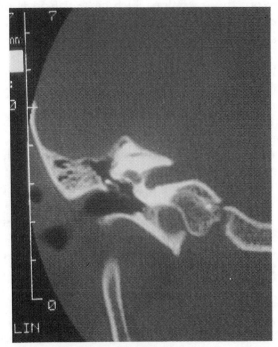

Figure 5.2 HRCT showing extensive new bone growth within the cochlear duct. (Courtesy of Drs Holland and Jaspan)

resultant increased risk of meningitis. Some surgeons would take the view in these cases that an extra-cochlear device is more appropriate in order to reduce or eliminate such risk. Other congenital abnormalities which may be detected include very narrow internal auditory meatus which might indicate a neural cause for the deafness caused by an absent eighth nerve (Shelton et al., 1989).

General medical assessment

Cochlear implantation in children requires at least one general anaesthetic, often two: one for the radiological investigation and one for the implantation operation itself. It is essential that each child is carefully assessed to ensure that he or she is fit enough to undergo such anaesthetic(s), bearing in mind that the surgery of implantation usually takes between 2 and 3 hours, and is likely to be longer if detailed electrophysiological and other recordings are carried out during the operation. This does not mean that children with other major system problems such as cardiovascular disease need to be excluded from consideration for implantation; it does mean that if such disease exists then it, in turn, must be expertly assessed in conjunction with a paediatric physician and also by the anaesthetist with whom the surgeon is going to carry out the operation. Such close liaison is inherent in all paediatric surgical practice and all paediatric otologists will be aware of the need for such cooperation.

It is not possible in a text such as this to cover all general medical possibilities but, if a practical and commonsense approach is taken, then even children with other significant pathology need not be denied the benefits of cochlear implantation.

A much more difficult area is to be found in the case of children with developmental delay; it is not possible in a text such as this to produce guidelines as individual circumstances vary so much. However, it is important to recognise the need for the individual child to be able to cooperate with the whole tuning and rehabilitation process, and the assessment will need to include reference to this area. As with general medical assessment, it may well prove necessary to liaise with a developmental paediatrician or paediatric neurologist.

Psychological assessment may be required but it is perhaps not necessary for all candidates for cochlear implantation to be formally examined by a paediatric psychologist, relying instead on the collective skills of the members of the cochlear implant team. The otologist(s) on the team will have a wide experience of paediatric medical practice and will bring this expertise to bear. If any suspicions are aroused, discussion will take place with the rehabilitation staff who similarly will have had great experience of the problems encountered by deaf children. If doubt still exists as to the suitability of an individual child, then formal psychological assessment may be required. In the case of a school-age child an educational psychologist's report may be available.

Of the children who have received implants in the Nottingham programme to date, only one has been deemed to need a formal psychological evaluation; it became apparent after implantation that in spite of excellent responses to sound stimulation this particular child, who had been deafened by meningitis, was not making appropriate and expected progress in the acquisition of speech. Psychological opinion suggested that he had developed a specific language disorder which had been revealed following implantation. This would have been impossible to predict before implantation.

Counselling

Counselling of parents of children who are candidates for implantation is an essential component of the preoperative work-up. It behoves all members of the team to be not only supportive of the parents but also to be realistic in the advice and counselling that they provide.

It is a legal obligation on any surgeon to ensure that the consent obtained for surgery is as fully informed as possible, that all questions have been properly answered and that the parents are aware of the risks of the surgery and possible complications as well as the benefits. The Appendix lists the risks and complications that need to be considered by parents before a decision is taken on implantation for their child.

It needs to be stressed to the parents that cochlear implantation is not just a surgical operation, but rather a long-term team effort involving great commitment by a large number of people interested in the general welfare of the child – this team includes the parents and extended family, school teachers and others in the school environment where this is appropriate, as well as many others who come into daily contact with the child. It is extremely helpful to the parents to have this information in written form and it is the practice at Nottingham to provide them with a booklet outlining these issues; this allows the parents the opportunity to reflect fully and comprehensively on discussions with them.

Particular sensitivity is required in dealing with the parents of children whose deafness has been acquired as a result of meningitis. Much, if not all, of their previous dealings with hospitals will have occurred during the particularly traumatic period of their child's illness with the meningitis which caused the deafness, and a frequent question such families raise is the possibility of the implant predisposing to further bouts of such infection. Firm reassurance is needed on this point.

Preoperative preparation

Once the decision to offer an implant has been taken, ratified at an implant team meeting, a date for surgery needs to be set and preparations made. There are many aspects of the preoperative period that are routine for any major operation and many of the points have already been covered. There must be no evidence of any intercurrent infection on admission for surgery. Typically cochlear implantation involves a 3–4 day stay in hospital and it is helpful if suitable facilities are available for the parents to stay during this time, either within the hospital itself or in nearby accommodation. The child may be helped to understand what is to happen by provision of a suitable booklet outlining in simple language and pictures an account of the operative period. Figure 5.3 shows such a booklet.

If the decision as to which ear is to be operated on has not already been taken on the basis of the audiological, radiological or otological assessment, then this will need to be finalised during the preoperative admission period, agreed with the parents and communicated to all concerned. It is the authors' belief that the child should be as aware as possible of what is going to happen while respecting the

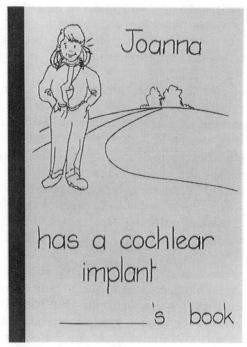

Figure 5.3 Information booklet for parents

views of the parents. A full explanation of the likely events during the postoperative period should be given and the parents should once again be given the opportunity to have any remaining questions answered. Other members of the implant team will often be able to provide further support at this stage. Finally the consent form should be formally signed by one of the parents or guardians.

The operation

On the morning of the operation the chld will be given anaesthetic pre-medication between 1 and 2 hours before being taken to the operating theatre. Usually one parent will accompany him or her to the anaes-thetic room and be permitted to stay until the child is unconscious.

Once the child is anaesthetised the head is shaved and he or she is then taken into the operating room itself. The operation is carried out through an incision as shown in Figure 5.4 and typically takes between 3 and 4 hours, including the time spent on carrying out measurement of stapedius reflex thresholds and recording electrically evoked brain-stem responses. The middle ear is approached through the mastoid antrum following which the inner ear is identified and a small opening fashioned for insertion of the electrode array which actually stimulates the nerve of hearing. Figure 5.5 shows a schema of the implant and

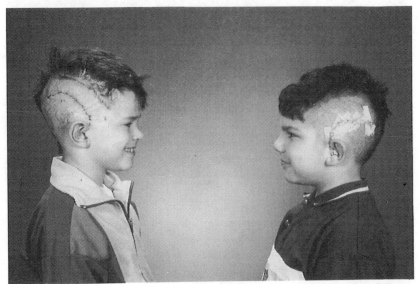

Figure 5.4 Two boys immediately after removal of the head dressing following cochlear implant surgery; note the incision used

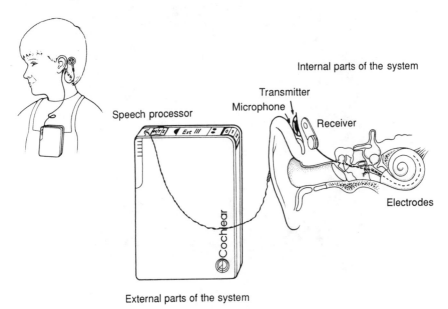

Figure 5.5 Schema of an intracochlear implant

Figure 5.6 is a picture of a boy wearing his implant. To avoid the need to remove sutures the wound is closed with absorbable stitches placed under the skin. A firm crêpe head bandage is placed on the head and left on for 2 days (Figure 5.7)

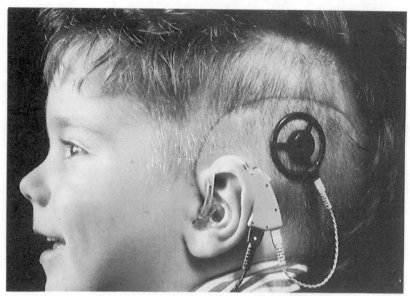

Figure 5.6 Patient HA wearing his processer for the first time

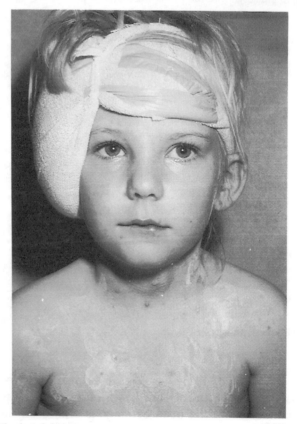

Figure 5.7 The head dressing

Postoperative care

Immediately following surgery, the child is brought to the recovery bay for initial postoperative care. The nurses in the recovery suite need to be reminded that the child is totally deaf and there is little point expecting a child either to respond to spoken requests or to be comforted by the usual phrases such as 'don't worry, your operation is all over', etc. It is the practice at Nottingham to ensure that at least one parent is escorted to the recovery area by a ward nurse so that a familiar face is there to greet the child as he or she surfaces from anaesthesia. This is an ideal time for the surgeon to explain to the parents the relevant details of the intervention; if electrophysiological tests have been satisfactorily undertaken, confirmation of the functional integrity of the system can be conveyed to the parents.

Communication

The surgeon should write to all professionals involved in the care of the child immediately following surgery. One can well understand the frustration local professionals experience if, having cared for a child over many years, they receive no direct communication about such a major event in the child's life. The communication need only be brief, outlining the type of implant used, the number of intracochlear channels inserted and any particular difficulties that were encountered. The local otolaryngologist will need to know if anything is expected of him or her – when the child ought to be seen and what care, if any, ought to be provided.

The implant warranty must be completed and returned to the manufacturer. It is important that patient confidentiality be respected when completing this documentation.

The surgeon also has the responsibility to remind parents about possible medical hazards associated with implantation. In particular, they should be reminded of the child's inability to have magnetic resonance imaging (MRI) and the harmful effects of monopolar diathermy at any site on the body. Some manufacturers provide a useful list in the implant package. It is the practice at Nottingham to offer all children a Medic Alert bracelet or necklace; this provides a telephone number, accessible 24 hours a day, to give key information to any physician who may be about to undertake emergency treatment of an implanted child.

Ward care

On return to the ENT children's ward, the child is usually drowsy and a firm pressure dressing surrounds the head, rather like a turban. The pressure dressing is aimed at preventing haematoma (a collection of blood clot) forming under the skin flap and is kept in place for 48 hours following surgery. An intravenous cannula is usually left in place for 24 hours to administer prophylactic antibiotics; after 24 hours, antibiotics are given orally and stopped after 3 days. The postoperative period is not particularly painful but may necessitate simple analgesic medication which should be given as frequently as is needed. By 24 hours following surgery, the child is usually mobile, and will have resumed a normal diet, albeit with some reluctance on occasions. Removal of the pressure dressing is greeted with relief and an opportunity to inspect the wound is taken.

The ward staff (kitchen staff and cleaners included) should be sensitive to the particular communication difficulties of the profoundly deaf child in the alien hospital environment. They should also be aware of the stress such surgery imposes on parents and their time may be needed to offer support. Above all, they should have a basic understanding of what is involved in cochlear implantation; the comments of a well-intentioned, but poorly informed, junior nurse or junior doctor can have devastating consequences for the emotionally charged parent. Professionals from the implant team should also try to visit the family during the period of hospitalisation; their visit can also serve to educate ward staff about implants.

Postoperative radiographs

Once the head dressing has been removed on either the second or third postoperative day, the child is brought to the radiology department for radiographs of the implant. A reversed Stenver's view is ideal and the view can be obtained without any special requirements, e.g. sedation. This radiograph (Figure 5.8) confirms satisfactory placement of the electrode bundle and allows the number of implanted electrodes to be counted (which can sometimes be difficult to do at the time of surgery). The radiograph is also useful as it provides a useful pictoral baseline of the implant which can be referred to in the future, especially if the child suffers a head injury or there is device failure. An experienced radiographer, who is prepared to communicate appropriately to the deaf child, is a great help.

Surgical outcome

Although a major surgical procedure on the ear, in experienced hands complications should be few. In the Nottingham series of 45 children (with an age range of 2;6–11;1 years) there were no significant early complications (haematoma, facial paralysis, wound infection, infection of the implanted device, vestibular disturbance, incorrect electrode placement, device extrusion, flap failure, etc.). In a multicentre series

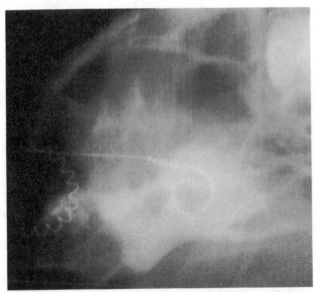

Figure 5.8 Postoperative radiograph showing full insertion of the intracochlear electrode array. (Courtesy of Drs Holland and Jaspan)

of 309 children implanted with the Nucleus 22 channel implant, the overall incidence of complications was 6.8%; major complications were more often reported in the smallest children (Clark, Cohen and Shepherd, 1991). Early in the Nottingham series one patient was found to have total bony obliteration of the labyrinth and the procedure was abandoned; it is now the practice at Nottingham to have a single-channel device available as a back-up to deal with such cases. The authors find that meticulous attention to detail (both in the soft tissue as well as the bony surgery) is an absolute imperative; if surgeons in training undertake implant surgery in young children, they should do so only under direct supervision if the incidence of complications is to be kept to a minimum.

Three of the children at Nottingham had late complications. One child developed pain on electrical stimulation; this child had complete bony obliteration and the only means of securing the electrode array was to drill a gutter in the promontory into which the electrodes were cemented; whether or not stimulation of the tympanic plexus caused the pain is uncertain, but this procedure which is unnecessarily destructive has now been abandoned. The second child developed a deep retraction pocket posterosuperiorly; the ear later discharged and exploration confirmed extensive cholesteatoma throughout the entire mastoid system, surrounding the electrode array. This child had two further explorations to control the disease, without any decrement in implant function. At the time of writing (December 1993) the child is awaiting a further exploration for suspected recurrent disease. In the third child a device failure occurred necessitating device removal; a further device was implanted uneventfully.

A continuing concern is the possibility of meningitis complicating otitis media in the implanted child. Animal studies have shown that the implant could indeed act as a conduit for the spread of infection from the middle ear to the labyrinth (Jackler, O'Donoghue and Schindler, 1986). However, many implanted children have developed otitis media and no documented case of meningitis acquired by a child in this way has been reported. Certainly, in the Nottingham series, the children who have developed otitis media have been treated in exactly the same way as non-implanted children with otitis media and there have been no complications.

A further concern is the issue of head growth and the possibility that increasing head expansion might distract the electrodes from within the cochlea. Although the cochlea attains full adult size before birth, the squamous, petrous, mastoid and tympanic portions of the temporal bone undergo considerable growth after birth. A number of studies have looked at the rate and size of the postnatal growth of the temporal bone (Eby and Nadol, 1986; O'Donoghue et al., 1986). An analysis of the postnatal growth of the temporal bone based on measurements of 103 CT scans of normal children revealed that 50% of the postnatal growth occurred in the first 2 years of life (O'Donoghue et al., 1986). The findings of Eby and Nadol (1986) based on plain skull radiographs are in agreement with these findings. This information would suggest that implantation might best be deferred until the age of 2 years which is consonant with current practice; this also allows time for the child to develop conditioning responses and for the family to come to terms with what deafness in childhood really means. There have been no reported cases of implant extrusion as a result of head growth alone but an expansile electrode array, which would accommodate head growth, would be ideal (O'Donoghue, Jackler and Schindler, 1986).

Conclusion

The decision to implant is an exercise in collective decision making by experienced professionals. The surgeon carries ultimate clinical responsibility for the care of the child and must be intimately involved in the decision making process. Above all, he or she must carefully counsel parents on all aspects of implantation, especially about their limitations and possible complications. The morbidity from cochlear implantation in young children is small provided it is undertaken by experienced surgeons. Complications will occur even in the most experienced hands but, while being disappointing, should not be disastrous if handled competently, expeditiously and sensitively.

An implant is for a child's life and should only be undertaken by those who have a genuine long-term professional commitment to these patients.

Appendix: risks/complications to be considered by parents

Infection:	this may need device removal.
Facial weakness:	this risk attends any ear surgery. Most causes of weakness following implantation are transient.
Balance symptoms:	usually transient.
Taste disturbance:	an uncommon complication for a few weeks following surgery.
Device failure:	the implanted electrodes may fail, but this is rare. The Nucleus device has received unconditional approval from the Food and Drug Administration in the USA for use in children. It is usually possible to replace device without any loss of functioning.
Risk of meningitis:	with middle-ear infection, this theoretical risk has not been borne out in practice.
Injury:	to any remaining sensory or neural tissue in the inner ear may occur from inserting the electrodes.
Electrochemical damage:	from long-term stimulation. The effects appear to be minimal based on current knowledge.
Need to remove the implant:	to allow for head growth or device failure. This has not been necessary in practice.
Limitation on certain activities:	that could damage or displace the device (e.g. rugby, boxing, squash). Swimming is possible if external parts are removed.
Note: only one ear will be implanted:	thus leaving the other ear available for futher developments.

The implant surgeons will be happy to provide information on any of the issues.

References

Bath, A.P., O'Donoghue, G.M., Holland, I.M. and Gibbin, K.P. (1994). Paediatric cochlear implantation: how reliable is computed tomography in assessing cochlear patency? *Clinical Otolaryngology* **18**, 475–479.

Eby T.L., Nadol J.B. 1986. Post natal growth of the human temporal bone. Implications for cochlear implants in children. *Annals of Otology, Rhinology and Laryngology* **95**, 356–364.

Clark, G.M., Cohen, N.L. and Shepherd, R.K. (1991). Surgical and safety considerations of multichannel cochlear implants in children. *Ear and Hearing* **12** (4), 15S–24S.

Gibbin K.P. 1992. Paediatric Cochlear Implantation. *Archives of Disease in Childhood.* **67**, 669–671.

Jackler R.K., O'Donoghue G.M., Schindler R.A. 1986. Cochlear implantation. Strategies to protect the implanted cochlea from middle ear infection.*Annals of Otology, Rhinology and Laryngology* **95**, 66–70.

Laszig, R, Terwey, B.., Battmer, R.D. and Hesse, G. 1988 Magnetic resonance imaging (MRI) and high resolution computertomography (HRCT) in cochlear implant candidates. *Scandinavian Audiology Supplementum (Copenhagen)* **30**, 197–200.

O'Donoghue G.M. (1992). Cochlear implants in children (Editorial). *Journal of the Royal Society of Medicine* **85**, 655–658.

O'Donoghue G.M., Jackler R.K., Schindler R.A. (1986) Observations on an experimental expansile electrode for use in cochlear implantation. *Acta OtoLaryngologica* **102**, 1–6.

O'Donoghue G.M., Jackler R.K., Jenkins W.M., Schindler R.A. (1986). Cochlear implantation in children: the problem of head growth. *Otolaryngology – Head and Neck Surgery* **94**, 78–81.

Shelton A, Luxford WM, Tonokawa L., Lo W.M., House W.F. 1989 The narrow internal auditory canal in children: a contraindication to cochlear implants. *Otolaryngology – Head and Neck Surgery* **100**, 227–231

Chapter 6
Electrophysiological tests

STEVE MASON

Cochlear implantation has now become an accepted approach to management of profoundly deafened children who obtain little or no benefit from conventional amplification (House, 1991; Miyamoto and Osberger, 1991; Staller, 1991). A paediatric cochlear implant programme for young children requires different professional skills and test techniques when compared to adult implantation (McCormick, 1991; Gibbin, 1992; O'Donoghue, 1992). Electrophysiological tests have a valuable role to play in the objective assessment of young children, both before and after implantation, using acoustical and electrical stimulation. The transfer from conventional acoustical stimulation of the cochlea to the electrical modality has led to the development of techniques for recording electrically evoked potentials (Miyamoto, 1986; Kileny, 1991; Shallop, 1993).

History

The functioning of the auditory system at different levels of the pathway has been extensively investigated in both humans and animals from recordings of electrical activity evoked by sounds. The electroencephalogram (EEG) was first recorded from the intact scalp in humans by Berger in 1929, and in the following year he described changes in the rhythm of the EEG to loud sounds (Berger, 1930). P.A. Davis (1939), and H. Davis and co-workers (1939) subsequently described more specific changes in the EEG. This was the birth of electric response audiometry (ERA). Development of appropriate technology and recording techniques has allowed the measurement of electrical responses to sound from the entire length of the auditory pathway (Picton et al., 1974; Abbas, 1988).

In 1957, Djourno and Eyries first reported a device which could

103

directly stimulate the cochlea and since then many investigators have studied the electrically generated sensation of hearing. Early studies of evoked potentials to electrical stimulation have been reported in both guinea-pigs (Meikle, Gillette and Godfrey, 1977; Gyo and Yanagihara, 1980) and humans (Starr and Brackmann, 1979). The requirement to have a method of objective evaluation of patients with cochlear implants has led to considerable interest in the application of electrically evoked potentials in the last few years. This is particularly relevant to the rapidly increasing number of young children receiving cochlear implants.

Evoked potentials

Recent reports have demonstrated that most types of auditory evoked potentials, similar to those associated with conventional ERA, can be recorded using electrical stimulation. These include the electrically evoked auditory brain-stem response, middle latency response and auditory cortical response (Pelizzone et al., 1989; Shallop et al., 1990; Kileny, 1991). Many of the advantages and drawbacks which affect the selection and application of a particular response are similar for both modes of stimulation. The auditory brain-stem response is therefore widely employed in young children for both acoustical and electrical stimulation. The recording techniques are similar for both modalities, although stimulus artefact is a specific technical difficulty which is encountered with electrical stimulation. Interpretation of the electrically evoked response requires a slightly different approach when compared to conventional ERA. Some of the amplitude and latency characteristics of the waveforms differ slightly from their acoustical counterpart, although the general morphology is often very similar. There is no basilar membrane travelling wave associated with generation of the electrically evoked potentials and the effects of this are most apparent on the brain-stem response.

Application

Electrophysiological tests in paediatric cochlear implantation have a role to play at various stages during selection of patients and after implantation, particularly in young children. Conventional ERA employing the auditory brain-stem response and occasionally electrocochleography is essential for objective confirmation of a profound hearing loss as part of the overall audiological assessment before implantation. Evoked potentials to electrical stimulation of the cochlea by the cochlear implant can be recorded during and after surgery, and provide a valuable objective measure of the functioning of the implant (Mason et al., 1993a; Shallop, 1993). The levels of electrical stimulation that a patient needs to perceive a stimulus can be predicted from recordings of the brain-stem response. This is particularly valuable for the initial fitting and tuning session in very young children when behavioural assessment can be difficult. The electrically evoked brain-stem response can also be recorded in the preoperative stage from electrical stimulation at the promontory or round window (Kileny et al., 1992a). This objective electrophysiological technique may have the ability to predict neuronal survival (Abbas and Brown, 1991).

There are two other objective techniques which are valuable for assessing cochlear implant function, the electrically evoked stapedius reflex (Battmer, Laszig and Lehnhardt, 1990; Stephan, Welze-Miller and Stiglbrunner, 1991) and the integrity test (Almqvist, Harris and Jonsson, 1993; Shallop, 1993). These techniques, although not strictly electrophysiological, are closely related in terms of their application. The threshold of the stapedius reflex is an indicator of the maximum comfortable levels of electrical stimulation that the patient might experience from the implant. The integrity test involves monitoring the stimulus artefact arising from the electrode array and thereby checks the functioning of the hardware and software of the implant system.

Electric response audiometry: pre-implant assessment

Electrical activity originating in the ear, auditory nerve and brain-stem pathways is known collectively as the early components of the auditory evoked potentials in ERA, and arises in the first 10 ms following an acoustical stimulus. These early components can be further subdivided into those arising from the cochlea and auditory nerve (electro-cochleography, ECochG), and those recorded predominantly from the brain-stem pathways (auditory brain-stem response). Response components in the subsequent 10–60 ms post-stimulus time period originate from the thalamus and primary auditory cortex (middle latency response, MLR) with later components representing activity from more general activation of secondary auditory cortex and frontal association cortex (auditory cortical response, ACR).

Paediatric electric response audiometry

The characteristics of the auditory brain-stem response and ECochG are most suited to application in paediatrics and have often been the preferred techniques for objective audiological assessment in young children. They are resilient to the effects of adaptation and habituation, and are not affected significantly by sleep, sedation or anaesthesia. In contrast the MLR and ACR can be very variable and unreliable in young children (Gibson, 1978; Stapells et al., 1988). The disadvantage of both the auditory brain-stem response and ECochG, however, is their limited ability to give precise information about hearing loss at specific frequencies of sound, particularly at mid to low tone frequency. The use of tone-pip stimuli as well as the click goes some way to improving the frequency specificity.

The auditory brain-stem response rather than ECochG is now preferred by many workers as an objective hearing test (H. Davis, 1976; Mokotoff, Schulman-Galambos and Galambos, 1977; Mason, McCormick and Wood, 1988). Historically, ECochG has been used extensively in both adults and children (Odenthal and Eggermont, 1974); however, electrode placement in both trans-tympanic and extra-tympanic methods in a young child usually requires a general anaesthetic. The availability of the simpler auditory brain-stem response technique, using surface scalp-recording electrodes, has largely superseded the routine use of ECochG except for special cases, as described later.

Auditory brain-stem response

The electrical activity evoked in the auditory nerve and brain-stem pathways by an auditory stimulus is known collectively as the auditory brain-stem response (ABR). The first definitive description of the ABR in humans was given by Jewett and Williston (1971), although Sohmer and Feinmesser first recorded these neurogenic responses in 1967. Jewett showed that the response evoked by a high-intensity click stimulus, and recorded from a vertex and ipsilateral mastoid electrode configuration, consists of a series of up to seven waves (designated I–VII in the Jewett classification), occurring in the first 10 ms after the stimulus (Figure 6.1). These waves are a far field recording of the electrical activity from sequentially activated neurons of the ascending auditory nerve and brain-stem pathways.

The precise origins of these waves are difficult to define and complicated by the interaction between different generator sites. Proposed origins are based largely on studies in animals (Achor and Starr, 1980), patients with brain-stem disorders (Stockard and Rossiter, 1977) or comparative studies of surface- and depth-recorded ABRs in patients undergoing surgery (Moller and Janetta, 1984). Wave I is known to be the compound action potential of the auditory nerve and is the far field equivalent of the action potential component in ECochG. Wave II is thought to arise predominantly from proximal regions of the auditory nerve and wave III from the cochlear nucleus. The superior olivary complex is considered to be the main source of wave IV and the lateral lemniscus wave V. Waves VI and VII are thought to arise mainly from the inferior colliculus. These proposed generator sites for waves II–VII are

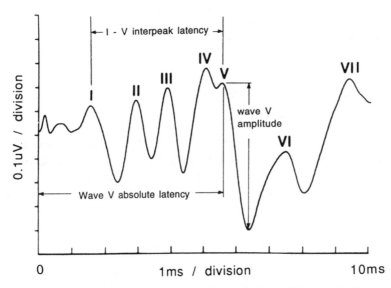

Figure 6.1 The waveform of the normal otoneurological ABR evoked by acoustical click stimulation with measurements of the amplitude and latency of waves I and V. (Adapted from Schwartz and Berry, 1985)

slightly more distal when compared to early studies of the ABR.

As well as these fast individual waves of the ABR, as described by Jewett and Williston, there is a slow wave associated with wave V and a negative component at a latency of about 10 ms. This slow negative response is often termed 'SN10' after Davis and Hirsh (1979) and is thought to originate in the mid-brain, probably representing post-synaptic activity within the inferior colliculus (Hashimoto, 1982). These slow components can be identified reliably with stimulus levels very close to hearing threshold as shown in Figure 6.2.

The stimulus and recording parameters for the ABR need to be selected to optimise the response characteristics and test procedure for either audiological application or as an otoneurological investigation. The slow components are recorded in the audiological ABR but only the fast waves for an otoneurological investigation. The appropriate test parameters for each type of application are well documented in the literature (Jacobson, 1985; Thornton, 1987; Mason, 1993; Lightfoot and Mason, 1993). A summary of typical values for the audiological ABR is as follows:

Electrode configuration:	active = vertex (Cz) or high forehead
	reference = ipsilateral mastoid
	guard = forehead or contralateral mastoid
Amplifier sensitivity:	typically 10 µV per display division
Artefact rejection level:	± 25 µV peak amplitude (referred to input)
On-line signal display	± 25 µV full scale

Filter bandwidth:	20 Hz (or 30 Hz) to 1 kHz (or 3 kHz)
Stimulus type:	click and tone pips (e.g. 1 kHz)
Stimulus polarity:	alternating phase
Repetition rate:	31 p.p.s.
Sweep time:	20 ms
Averaging sweeps:	2000
Averaged display:	± 1 µV full scale
Plotter output:	0.2 µV/ cm

The averaged display and plotter output values are typical for a response evoked by a 60 dB nHL stimulus in normal hearing. Small responses which may be encountered in pre-implant assessment may require an increase by a factor of two in sensitivity for the display and

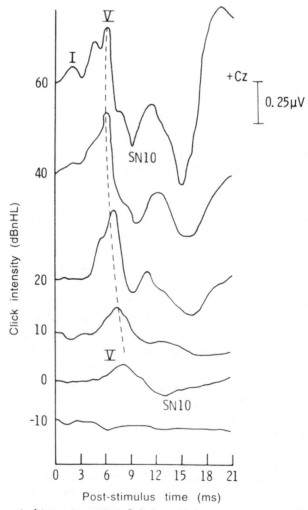

Figure 6.2 A typical intensity series of click-evoked audiological ABR waveforms in normal hearing

plot. However, care must be taken to avoid the mistaken identification of noise for a response in this situation, and any possible small response component must be confirmed by appropriate replication of the waveform. The stimulus is normally presented to the patient through standard Telephonics-type headphones. Electric and magnetic screening of these headphone transducers, using mu-metal enclosures, can be helpful in reducing the effects of artefacts arising from high-intensity stimuli. Other methods of stimulus presentation such as bone conduction (Schwartz and Berry, 1985) and via a hearing aid (Mahoney, 1985) are available, but these techniques can degrade the effectiveness of the stimulus in generating a well-defined response waveform and are difficult to implement at high intensity levels.

The following test parameters are changed from the audiological settings to optimise the ABR for an otoneurological investigation.

Electrode configuration:	active = vertex (Cz)
	reference = ipsilateral mastoid/earlobe
	guard = forehead or contralateral mastoid
Filter bandwidth:	100 Hz to 3 kHz
Stimulus type:	click only
Stimulus polarity:	alternating phase (occasionally single phase)
Repetition rate:	11 p.p.s.
Sweep time:	12 ms

The three major changes involve the low frequency cut-off of the filter, a slower stimulus repetition rate and a shorter sweep time. These changes all enhance the identification of the faster waveform components (waves I, III and V) and improve the accuracy of the latency measurements which are required for an otoneurological investigation.

Electrocochleography

Three response components are recorded in ECochG: cochlear microphonics (CM), summating potential (SP) and the compound auditory nerve action potential (AP). The CM and SP are predominantly receptor potentials, and reflect the functional status of the hair cells. The AP is the summation of electrical activity from a large number of individual nerve fibres originating from close to the cochlea. The AP is the only component of ECochG which has good threshold sensitivity and can be used for assessment of hearing threshold. Typical recordings of the different components in ECochG are shown in Figure 6.3. There are two commonly used locations for the recording electrode in ECochG. The trans-tympanic method, first described by Portmann, Lebert and Aran in 1967, involves the placing of a needle electrode through the tympanic membrane coming to rest on the promontory in the middle ear. This technique gives a large well-defined response, but is

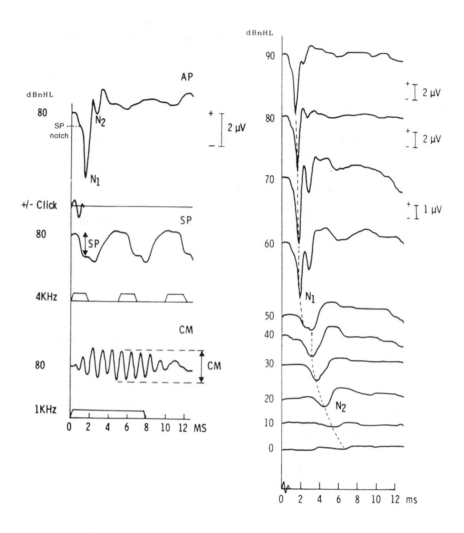

Figure 6.3 Extra-tympanic electrocochleography in the normal ear showing the three response components: the compound auditory nerve action potential (AP), summating potential (SP) and cochlear microphonics (CM). Only the AP can be recorded reliably with stimulus levels close to threshold

invasive and requires a general anaesthetic in children. An alternative method is the extra-tympanic technique which involves positioning an electrode in the external auditory meatus close to the tympanic membrane (Mason, Singh and Brown, 1980). This technique is non-invasive and can be used more readily in older children and adults than the trans-tympanic method. However, in young children this technique still requires a general anaesthetic. A more detailed discussion of the recording techniques and clinical application of ECochG can be found in Gibson (1978) and Abramovich (1990). A summary of appropriate stimulus and recording parameters is as follows:

Electrode configuration:	active = (a) ear canal for extra-tympanic (XECochG)
	(b) promontory for trans-tympanic (TECochG)
	reference = ipsilateral earlobe
	guard = forehead
Amplifier sensitivity:	typically 10 µV or 20 µV per display division
Artefact rejection level:	± 50 µV peak amplitude (referred to input)
On-line signal display:	± 50 µV full scale
Filter bandwidth:	30 Hz to 3 kHz
Stimulus type:	click and tone pip (e.g. 500 Hz, 1 kHz)
Stimulus polarity:	single phases with waveform subtraction for the CM alternating phase for the SP/AP waveform
Repetition rate:	11 p.p.s.
Sweep time:	10 ms
Averaging sweeps:	2000 (XECochG), 500 (TECochG)
Averaged display:	± 3 µV full scale (XECochG), ± 30 µV full scale (TECochG)
Plotter output:	0.5 µV/ cm (XECochG), 5 µV/ cm (TECochG)

The averaged display and plotter output values are typical for a response evoked by a 60 dB nHL stimulus in normal hearing. An increase in sensitivity by a factor of two or four may be required to assist identification of a small response. The ECochG stimulus is usually presented to the patient through a mu-metal shielded Telephonics-type headphone to achieve reliable differentiation of true CM from stimulus artefact.

Clinical application

In young children who are possible candidates for cochlear implantation, ERA must be carried out as part of the overall audiological assessment to confirm a profound hearing loss. The ABR and ECochG are the most appropriate responses to employ for this investigation and either one can be used to support the audiological diagnosis. The simpler electrode procedure for the ABR is attractive when compared with ECochG and is now the technique most often preferred.

Stimulus

The click stimulus is widely used in ERA and provides valuable information regarding hearing in the 2–4 kHz region of the audiogram (Drift, Brocaar and van Zanten, 1987). However, the status of hearing at lower tone frequencies than the click is very important because residual hearing is more likely to be present towards the left-hand side of the audiogram in potential cochlear implant candidates. The use of mid to low frequency tone-pip stimuli (typically 500 Hz and 1 kHz) provides valuable additional information from the ABR and ECochG investigation. The evoked potential generated by these tone-pip stimuli, however, does have limited frequency specificity, particularly with high intensity levels, as a result of the spread of energy in the cochlea away from the nominal tone frequency (Stapells et al., 1985). Nevertheless, any residual cochlear activity in the region of the tone-pip frequency should evoke a detectable response. Loss of frequency specificity is usually a result of electrical activity being generated from more basal regions of the cochlea than the tone-pip frequency. Profound hearing loss at high frequency effectively stops the cochlea from responding and, to some extent, improves the overall frequency specificity of the response evoked by a mid to low frequency tone-pip stimulus. Ipsilateral high-pass masking can be used to improve the frequency specificity but this is at the expense of a reduction in the ability to detect a response.

Test protocol

A test protocol for pre-implant ERA assessment which includes both click and tone-pip stimuli is employed in the Nottingham Paediatric Cochlear Implant Programme. Each child has an ERA assessment on both ears usually carried out as the final stage of the audiological work-up. The routine protocol employs the ABR using click and tone-pip (500 Hz and 1 kHz) stimuli with intensity levels up to 105 dB nHL. This is around the maximal intensity level which can be achieved with transient stimuli and is limited by the maximum peak sound pressure level that can be generated by the headphone. The ABR is recorded as an audiological assessment using three stimuli (click, 500 Hz and 1 kHz tone-pips) and as an otoneurological investigation with a high intensity click stimulus. This protocol takes about 60 minutes to complete and a young child (typically less than 5 years) usually requires sedation to achieve a quiet signal baseline for this length of time. The child is sedated on the ENT ward and the ABR investigation carried out in a quiet sideroom. In a slightly older cooperative child it may be possible to carry out the investigation without sedation, with the child lying on a couch or bed. Reliable recordings of residual responses, particularly to mid and low frequency tone-pips, does require a very low noise baseline signal.

Electrocochleography is kept in reserve for special cases in the Nottingham pre-implant assessment protocol. This situation may arise if there are ambiguous findings between the behavioural and ABR assessment, or if the possibility of a progressive, fluctuating or retrocochlear deafness exists. A recording of the summating potential component of ECochG can be useful in this situation to assess the presence of endolymphatic hydrops. In a child with persistent conductive hearing loss, who is already having a general anaesthetic for removal of middle-ear glue and insertion of grommets, the opportunity should be taken to carry out either ECochG or ABR immediately after surgery while the child is still anaesthetised. This will help to minimise the effects of conductive loss on the outcome of the ERA investigation. Unfortunately the outcome of the ERA appears to be slightly complicated in some cases as a result of an apparent transient threshold shift originating from the surgical procedure. Interpretation of the ERA should allow for the possibility of this effect being present.

Tympanograms should be recorded whenever possible at the time of ERA to check for good middle-ear function and to exclude the possible effects of a conductive hearing loss on the outcome of ERA (Finitzo-Hieber and Friel-Patti, 1985). A true measure of sensorineural hearing loss with acoustical stimuli is not possible if a flat compliance is recorded, which may necessitate a repeat ERA test. Exclusion and management of middle-ear pathology is therefore essential before audiological and ERA assessment. The intensity which can be achieved with a bone-conduction stimulus is limited and is inappropriate for assessment of profound sensorineural hearing loss in the pre-implant evaluation.

Typical outcome

The acoustical ERA investigation is used to confirm a profound hearing loss which is already strongly suspected from subjective and behavioural audiological assessment. The most common outcome is therefore an absence of all response components, or occasionally some residual response activity, as shown in Figure 6.4a. Reliable interpretation of this condition requires at least two averaged waveforms to check for repeatability of any possible small response components. Identification of significant levels of response activity on one or both ears is important because this may influence the decision of which ear to implant or, in some cases, suggest further audiological assessment before proceeding with implantation. Many young children being implanted have acquired a profound hearing loss from meningitis. Some recovery of hearing loss after meningitis has been reported (McCormick et al., 1993) and therefore any response activity on ERA should be examined carefully to exclude, as far as possible, any improvement in hearing. The ear with least or no response to acoustical stimulation is usually chosen for implantation providing there are no other contraindications such as ossification of the cochlea.

In children where a reliable ABR waveform is recorded the threshold of the response must be measured. The otoneurological ABR should also be recorded to attempt a measurement of the absolute

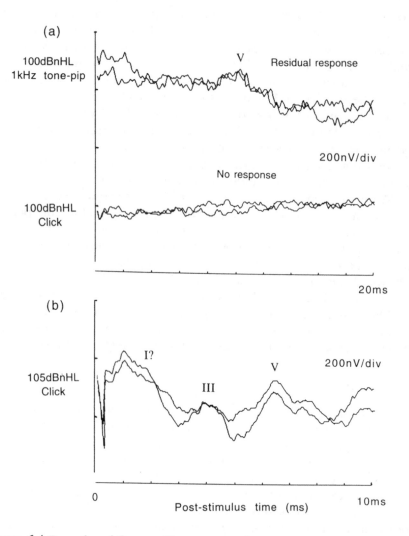

Figure 6.4 Examples of the possible outcome of a pre-implant ERA assessment from (a) audiological and (b) otoneurological recordings of the ABR. A no response condition is most common with the occasional presence of a residual response. Identification of a possible wave I, wave III and V is indicated in (b). In this example, the latency measurements were considered to be just within the limits of the normal range for a young child with severe hearing loss

latency and interpeak latency values of waves I, III and V (Figure 6.4b). A normal wave I–V interpeak interval will help to exclude retrocochlear pathology which might restrict the performance of the implant. An absence of all response components on the ABR waveform (including wave I) is consistent with cochlear hearing loss, but cannot exclude the possibility of retrocochlear pathology or neural damage.

Electrically evoked potentials

The introduction of the technique for recording electrically evoked potentials in the field of cochlear implantation has provided a valuable tool for the objective assessment of response to electrical stimulation. Early clinical experience with cochlear prostheses has been achieved with a postlingually deafened adult population using relatively simple devices. However, an increase in the sophistication of implants, and their wider application in the congenitally deaf and paediatric population in whom prior experience with sound may be limited or lacking, has generated a need for electrophysiological tests to determine the functional state of a cochlear implant.

Types of response

Electrical stimulation of the cochlea evokes neural activity in the ascending auditory pathway which can be recorded using techniques similar to those employed in conventional acoustical ERA. The different classes of electrically evoked potentials are directly related to their acoustical counterparts to the extent that similar terminology is often applied with a leading 'E' to denote the electrical response. The range of responses reported in the literature includes the electrically evoked action potential (EAP), auditory brain-stem response (EABR), middle latency response (EMLR), auditory cortical response (EACR) and cognitive potentials. Many of the waveform components within each type of electrically evoked response are thought to arise from similar generator sites as in acoustical stimulation.

Electrically evoked action potential

The EAP has been successfully recorded from humans by Brown and Abbas (1990) using different channels of an Ineraid intracochlear electrode array for electrical stimulation and recording the response. A subtraction technique was used to extract the response component from the stimulus artefact. This method of recording the EAP is technically difficult and is dependent on having direct access to the intracochlear electrodes through the percutaneous connector of the Ineraid device. The EAP waveform described by Brown and Abbas consists of a predominantly negative deflection at approximately 0.4 ms after onset of the current stimulus. They postulate that the peripheral EAP response may be more directly related to neuronal survival than the more centrally derived EABR. Unfortunately implementation of this method of recording the EAP is not possible in devices such as the Nucleus Mini System 22 and the MED-EL broadband analogue implant which use a radiofrequency (RF) transcutaneous transmission system.

Electrically evoked auditory brain-stem response

The typical waveform characteristics of the EABR evoked by an intra-cochlear electrical pulse stimulus can be seen in Figure 6.5a and are generally similar to the acoustical ABR (Abbas and Brown, 1991). However, there are some important differences particularly with respect to the latency of the response, with components arising around 1 to 1.5 ms earlier for the EABR compared with the ABR (Allum et al., 1990). The lack of cochlear mechanics with electrical stimulation, such as the travelling wave along the basilar membrane, is one reason for the shorter latency. The individual components of the EABR waveform are thought to have similar generator sites to the ABR (Pelizzone, Kasper and Montandon, 1989) and are often denoted by a leading 'e' applied to the standard waves of the acoustic ABR, for example eV. With high intensity stimuli it is possible to identify most of the 'e' waves normally seen in the ABR except for wave eI which is almost always obscured by the stimulus artefact. The wave eV component is generally used to identify response threshold.

Electrically evoked middle latency response

Response activity in the thalamic auditory pathway and primary auditory cortex, evoked by electrical stimulation, is known as the electrically evoked middle latency response (EMLR). The most prominent components of the EMLR are eNa, ePa and eNb (Figure 6.5b) and can be recorded reliably in adult subjects (Kileny, 1991). These three components arise in the latency period from about 25 to 35 ms and are slightly earlier than their acoustical counterpart (Kileny, Kemink and Miller, 1989). One advantage of recording these response components compared to the EABR is that there is minimal spread of stimulus artefact into this later time period. The consistency of the EMLR, is however, dependent on the psychological state of the patient in the same way as the acoustical MLR. Application of this response is therefore restricted in young children, particularly during sedation and general anaesthesia. Early attempts at recording electrically evoked potentials were more successful with the EMLR (Shallop et al., 1990) until the technique for the EABR had been refined.

Electrically evoked auditory cortical response

Electrical stimulation of the cochlea will evoke activity in the auditory pathway which subsequently generates a response at cortical level (Brix and Gedlicka, 1991; Kileny, 1991). This high level response is termed the 'electrically evoked auditory cortical response' (EACR) and has similar characteristics to the acoustic ACR. The eN1 component at a latency of about 100 ms and an eP2 at 150–200 ms are the most prominent

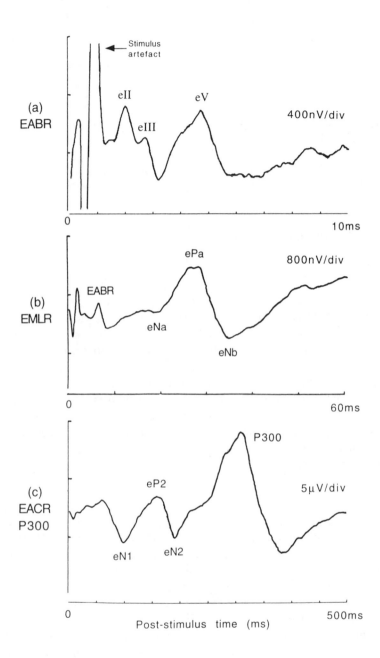

Figure 6.5 Typical response waveforms evoked by electrical stimulation using an intracochlear electrode including (a) the electrically evoked auditory brain-stem response, (b) middle latency response (adapted from Shallop et al., 1990), (c) cortical responses (adapted from Kileny, 1991), and (d) mismatch negativity. The MMN waveform has been elicited by the difference in response to standard (common) and deviant (rare) speech stimuli. (Adapted from Kraus et al., 1992)

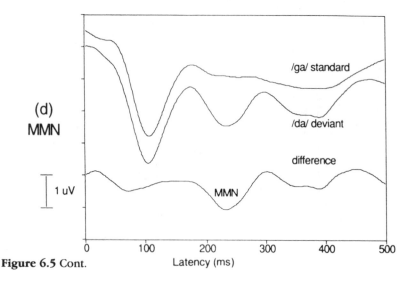

Figure 6.5 Cont.

elements of the adult response. The response is inconsistent in young children, particularly during sleep, sedation and general anaesthesia, and this is probably the reason why there are so few reports of paediatric applications of the EACR. In awake older children (aged 10 years or more) and adults the EACR is much more consistent and reliable (Figure 6.5c). The whole auditory pathway can be assessed and problems of contamination of the signal baseline with stimulus artefact are minimal. Characteristics of this high level cortical response in conjunction with slightly later cognitive potentials may, in the future, provide an insight into the processing and recognition of patterns of electrical stimulation arising from environmental sounds and speech.

Cognitive potentials

Event related potentials associated with cognition of an acoustical signal, such as the mismatch negativity (MMN) and the P300 (Regan, 1989; Taylor, 1991; Kraus et al., 1992), have been recorded in both adults and children. These responses can be elicited by means of an oddball paradigm involving the infrequent presentation of rare (target) stimuli interspersed within more frequent common (non-target) stimuli. The MMN is the difference in the cortical activity elicited by these two stimuli and is most dominant at a latency of around 200 ms. It is a passive response and does not require active attention to the stimuli. The P300 is an endogenous cortical response with a latency of around 300 ms which is enhanced by attending to the rare (target) stimuli. The amplitude and latency characteristics of the P300 are highly dependent on age, mental status, expectation and the degree of difficulty of the test paradigm.

The MMN and P300 can be elicited by electrical stimulation in patients with cochlear implants (Oviatt and Kileny, 1991; Kraus et al., 1993). Typical response waveforms are shown in Figure 6.5c. The configuration of the MMN evoked by speech stimuli presented through an implant was reported to be remarkably similar to the response measured in normally hearing adult subjects (Kraus et al., 1993). The electrically evoked P300 tended to exhibit a longer latency than the equivalent acoustically generated response (Kileny, 1991). Kileny speculated that this difference resulted from the increased difficulty of the task for cochlear implant recipients, or that it reflected overall slower auditory processing as a result of previous auditory deprivation before implantation. The MMN and P300 in cochlear implant recipients show promise as objective measures of discrimination ability, and for the study of central auditory processing.

Electrically evoked auditory brain-stem response in young children

The characteristics and behaviour of responses such as the EABR, EMLR and EACR are very similar to their equivalent acoustical response, particularly during sleep, sedation and general anaesthesia. It is not surprising therefore that the EABR has received the widest development and application in the paediatric population analogous to the ABR in conventional ERA. The response is very robust for the effects of the psychological state of the patient, which satisfies the requirements of an objective tool for use in young children.

The EABR can provide information about the functioning of a cochlear implant, including a prediction of the level of electrical stimulation required for subjective perception of the stimulus. Intraoperative recordings of the EABR at the time of implant surgery is a popular test protocol (Shallop et al., 1991; Mason et al., 1993a) which takes advantage of the child already being anaesthetised. Amplitude of the EABR is very small close-to-threshold and the test technique is best suited to the quiet recording conditions which a general anaesthetic can offer. The EABR is as an essential facility in a paediatric cochlear implant programme, with other types of electrically evoked potentials, such as the MMN and P300, potentially valuable for the future.

Recording technique for the electrically evoked auditory brain-stem response

Many aspects of the recording technique for the EABR are similar to those for the acoustical response, employing well-established methodology and technology. The major difference is the way in which the stimulus is delivered to the ear and the resultant activation of nerve fibres. Artefacts arising from this stimulus are the main technical difficulty associated with recording the EABR. These artefacts arise from the electrical component of the stimulus as well as the RF transcutaneous transmission signal, which is employed in implant devices such as the Nucleus Mini System 22 and the MED-EL broadband analogue system.

Delivery of the stimulus is often via the intracochlear electrode array of the implant, although extracochlear techniques at the promontory and round window can also be employed. In paediatric application an intracochlear implant with a RF transcutaneous transmission system is normally preferred, in contrast to those with a percutaneous plug connection such as the Ineraid device. A general description of the EABR test technique will be presented. This will also be supported by a slightly more detailed discussion of the Nucleus system which is a popular choice for use in young children.

Instrumentation

A schematic diagram of the instrumentation required for eliciting and recording the EABR is shown in Figure 6.6 and can be conveniently described in two parts. An implant system is often used to generate and present the electrical stimulus to the ear, and an evoked potential system records the response. These two components of the system must be accurately linked in time via a trigger pulse so that data collection is synchronised with onset of the stimulus. Most implant systems now have a trigger pulse available for this purpose which can be applied to an external trigger input on the evoked potential system. However, the triggering edge of this pulse that the recording equipment recognises, which may be either the positive or negative going phase, may have an inherent offset in time from the onset of the stimulus. A correction for this difference in timing should be applied to latency measurements of the EABR to achieve a true absolute value.

Unfortunately, programming software which has been originally designed for controlling the presentation of the stimulus during fitting and tuning of the implant is not always the most appropriate for EABR

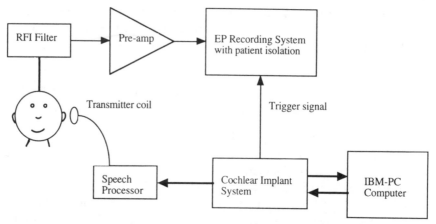

Figure 6.6 A schematic diagram of instrumentation for recording the EABR

application. The technique ideally requires a train of stimuli (e.g. biphasic pulses) where the repetition rate, intensity and onset polarity can be controlled. Manufacturers are now becoming more aware of some of these stimulus requirements and are incorporating them in current software developments.

Delivery of the stimulus

The electrical stimulus is delivered either through a single channel of an intracochlear electrode array in the scala tympani or with an extra-cochlear electrode positioned on the promontory or round window. Extracochlear stimulation is usually employed in preoperative assessment or with a single-channel implant where it is not possible to introduce an intracochlear electrode array as a result of ossification or deformity of the cochlea. A subjective response to extracochlear preoperative stimulation is employed in adult subjects to assist the selection of patients for implantation and to assess the potential performance of an implant (Gray and Baguley, 1990; Kilney et al., 1992b). In young children there are obvious difficulties with cooperation and implementation of this behavioural technique, and electrode placement requires a general anaesthetic. A recording of the EABR evoked by electrical stimulation can be employed as an objective promontory test. Kileny et al. (1992a) have taken the opportunity to carry out this investigation immediately before implant surgery begins, after the child has been anaesthetised, to establish the ear which responds best to electrical stimulation.

Stimulus characteristics

The most commonly used stimulus to evoke the EABR is a bipolar electrical pulse. This type of stimulus has an almost instantaneous rise and fall time, and short duration (typically 200–400 µs). These timing characteristics are very similar to the electrical pulse used to generate the acoustical click stimulus and has a very high level of synchronisation of neural activity which is optimum for eliciting the EABR. A train of individual bipolar pulses are required in order to complete a recording of an averaged waveform consisting of 1000 or 2000 sweeps. A number of different repetition rates for the stimulus (interstimulus interval) have been used ranging from 10 p.p.s. (Shallop et al., 1991) up to 85 p.p.s. (Mason et al., 1993b). There is less adaptation of the individual waves of the EABR with electrical stimulation compared with the acoustic ABR. The adaptive mechanisms in the cochlea involved with generation of the acoustic ABR are bypassed with electrical stimulation. There is advantage in using a relatively fast stimulus rate (typically 31 p.p.s. or higher) to reduce the test time. The maximum length sequence (MLS) technique for data collection with very fast stimulus rates, which has been investigated with acoustical stimuli (Picton, Champagne and Kellett, 1992), may have useful application in the recording of the EABR.

The intensity or loudness of the stimulus perceived by the patient is dependent on electric charge which is related to the amplitude of the current (or voltage) and the duration of the stimulus (e.g. pulse width). In many implant systems, stimulus intensity is expressed in arbitrary units such as 'stimulus units' (0–239) for the Nucleus implant and 'dBV' (–60 to +10) for the MED-EL device. For an intracochlear electrode the delivered charge is typically in the range 10–200 nanocoloumbs (nC) for most implant users which is equivalent to 50 μA to 1 mA for a pulse duration of 200 μs.

A train of electrical pulses for eliciting the EABR can be delivered by the Nucleus implant system with the mini speech processor (MSP) using appropriate selection of stimulus parameters in the programming software (DPS). A sufficient number of bursts of stimulus pulses to complete an averaged waveform (2000 sweeps) are generated by selecting a 1000 ms pulse duration and 1 ms interstimulus interval, and entering a 99 G command from the keyboard. The pulse rate of the stimuli within the train can be selected and is typically in the range 31–85 p.p.s. for the EABR compared to 250 or 500 p.p.s. for subjective threshold measurements of the stimulus during tuning (T levels). A minimum of 15 p.p.s. is recommended by Cochlear Corporation so that sufficient power transfer by the RF transcutaneous transmission system is achieved during periods of stimulation. The electrical pulse stimulus can be generated in either a stimulus or current mode. Intensity in stimulus mode is controlled by changes in both the width of the pulse and current amplitude, whereas in current mode only changes in amplitude of current are employed. Tuning and use of the implant are usually implemented in stimulus mode and therefore measurements of the EABR with the same mode will be compatible with subjective assessments. Stimuli can be presented on a selected channel of the electrode array (active) with a reference provided by other single electrodes (bipolar, BP) or multiple electrodes across the array (common ground, CG). A typical intensity series of EABR waveforms for the Nucleus implant are shown in Figure 6.7 using stimulus mode with a CG reference and a pulse rate of 31 p.p.s. Best definition of the EABR waveform is often observed from stimulation of the more apical electrode channels, e.g. channel 20.

Recording methodology

Most commercially available evoked potential (EP) systems are suitable for recording the EABR providing that a trigger pulse from the implant

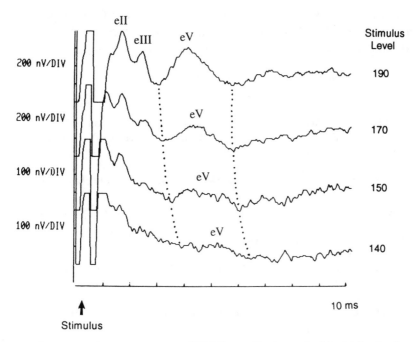

Figure 6.7 A typical intensity series of EABR waveforms evoked by biphasic electrical pulses presented on channel 20 of the Nucleus electrode array. The most dominant components of the waveform are often waves eII, eIII and eV

equipment can be interfaced to an external trigger input on the EP system. The on-going EEG signal is recorded from standard silver/silver chloride scalp electrodes positioned at the vertex (active) and mastoid (reference) with a guard electrode on the forehead. For intraoperative recordings of the EABR the contralateral mastoid is often employed as a convenient reference site rather than the conventional ipsilateral site. The contact impedance of each electrode should always be less than 4 kΩ. Amplifier sensitivity is normally set to around 10 or 20 µV per division with artefact rejection disabled across the time period of the stimulus artefact (typically 0–2 ms) otherwise there will be rejection of the signal. The EABR is often recorded with an amplifier filter bandwidth of 100Hz–3000 Hz. There is no evidence of slow components associated with the wave eV in the EABR, which are normally observed in the acoustic ABR, and therefore there is no advantage in using a low cut-off frequency which extends down to 20 or 30 Hz (Mason, 1984). A post-stimulus epoch of 10 ms is adequate to capture the response waveform because there is only a small increase in wave eV latency with reduction in stimulus intensity. Signal averaging of 2000 individual sweeps, in conjunction with appropriate replication of the averaged waveform, is essential for reliable identification of small responses close-to-threshold. However, at high suprathreshold levels there is often a rapid growth in response amplitude and 1000 sweeps may be sufficient for reliable identification of the response waveform. A summary of stimulus and recording parameters for the EABR is as follows:

Electrode configuration:	active = vertex (Cz)
	reference = contralateral mastoid
	guard = forehead
Amplifier sensitivity:	10 µV or 20 µV per display division
Artefact rejection level:	± 25 µV peak amplitude (referred to input signal)
On-line signal display:	± 25 µV full scale
Filter bandwidth:	100 Hz to 3 kHz
Stimulus type:	biphasic electrical pulse (typically 200–400 µs per phase)
Stimulus polarity:	ideally alternating onset phase to reduce stimulus artefact
Pulse rate:	typically 31 p.p.s.
Sweep time:	10 ms
Averaging sweeps:	2000 (1000 with high suprathreshold stimuli)
Averaged display:	± 1 µV full scale (± 5 µV with high suprathreshold stimuli)
Plotter output:	0.2 µV/ cm (1 µV with high suprathreshold stimuli)

Stimulus artefact

The main difficulty in recording a high-quality EABR waveform arises from contamination of the signal with artefacts associated with presentation of the stimulus. These artefacts originate from the electrical stimulus and from RF interference in the case of a transcutaneous transmission implant system such as the Nucleus and MED-EL devices. The RF component of the artefact can be removed by placing a passive RF filter in line with the electrode leads (Game, Thomson and Gibson, 1990; Mason et al., 1993a) but this will still leave the electrical component of the artefact. Amplitude of the electrical artefact depends on the intensity of the stimulus and can sometimes interfere with the response waveform at high stimulus levels. The preamplifier and main amplifier need to be able to handle this artefact in terms of having relatively quick recovery from possible saturation at the onset of the trace. Recording the signal with a very low cut-off frequency (typically 1 Hz) on the filter bandwidth can be helpful in reducing the spread of a large artefact across the EABR waveform. Some workers have employed a signal blanking circuit across the time period of the stimulus artefact (Millard, McAnally and Clark, 1992). The electrical component of the artefact is generally larger with extracochlear stimulation compared with intracochlear, because of the effects of current spread, and presents greater problems in recording a good quality EABR.

Contamination of the averaged EABR waveform by the electrical component of the stimulus artefact can be reduced by presenting a train of stimulus pulses where the onset polarity is alternately inverted; this is analogous to the alternately inverted click stimulus in the acoustical domain. During the averaging process this will result in significant cancellation of the artefact. Unfortunately a biphasic pulse with alternating onset phase is not readily available on commercially available implant systems.

Intraoperative test procedure

The use of an intraoperative test procedure for recording the EABR in young children takes advantage of the child already being anaesthetised for implant surgery. This is a popular test protocol and has been adopted in the Nottingham programme for the multichannel Nucleus implant and more recently the MED-EL single-channel extracochlear device. Attachment of the scalp-recording electrodes is normally carried out in the operating room immediately after administration of the general anaesthetic and before the child is prepared for surgery. Electrode leads are colour-coded for future reference as access to the scalp is not practical during the operation. After implantation of the electrode array and receiver, the transmitter coil and lead are placed in a sterile clear plastic sheath (40 mm x 1 m) and positioned over the receiver in the wound. The EABR is recorded with a range of electrical stimulus levels on electrode channels 20, 15, 10 and 5. The stimulus level is changed in steps of 20 stimulus units at high suprathreshold levels and in steps of 10 units close-to-threshold. Response threshold of the wave eV component of the EABR is then estimated to the nearest 5 units by interpolation. The recording procedure is completed in about 20–30 minutes during closure of the wound and suturing of the skin flap, and requires very little additional time in the operating room. The electrically evoked stapedius reflex is also recorded during the operation just before the EABR measurements (Sheppard et al., 1992).

Current application of the electrically evoked auditory brain-stem response

Application of electrically evoked potentials in patients receiving cochlear implants, and in particular the EABR in young children, is an exciting and relatively new development in the field of electrophysiological testing. Electrical stimulation of the cochlea and subsequent functioning of the auditory pathway can be assessed using the EABR and is complemented by other objective methods such as the electrically evoked stapedius reflex and integrity testing.

Interpretation of the response waveform

Intracochlear stimulation usually evokes an EABR which has more clearly defined waveform characteristics compared to the response from an extracochlear stimulus. The basic features of the response are, however, similar for both methods of electrical stimulation. All the individual components of the EABR arise earlier than their equivalent counterparts in the acoustic ABR and this must be taken into consideration regarding interpretation of the waveform. The absolute latency of wave eV arises at around 4.0–4.5 ms compared with 5.5–6.0 ms for the acoustical wave V. Wave eV is usually the component examined for estimation of response threshold, although in some implanted patients waves II and III are equally dominant close-to-threshold. Amplitude of wave eV is determined in a similar way to the acoustical ABR using a peak-to-trough measurement.

In addition to the neurogenic components of the EABR, a compound muscle action potential is occasionally seen in some patients particularly with extracochlear stimulation. Excessive spread in current can cause direct stimulation of other neural pathways such as the facial nerve (Muller-Deile, Schmidt and Rudert, 1993). These muscle responses are relatively large when compared to the EABR.

Typical changes in amplitude and latency of wave eV with stimulus intensity (I/O functions) are shown in Figure 6.8. There is only a small increase in latency with reduction in stimulus level. The amplitude I/O function is shallow close-to-threshold but becomes very steep with increases in stimulus intensity at high suprathreshold levels. Amplitude of the wave eV component often rises from around 50 nV at response threshold up to 1 μV or more with high levels of electrical stimulation.

Functioning of the cochlear implant

Electrically evoked auditory brain-stem response

The presence of an EABR waveform confirms that the auditory nerve fibres are receiving and reacting to electrical stimulation, and response activity is being generated in the brain-stem pathways. This technique is therefore an excellent check of the functioning of both the hardware of the implant system and the physiological status of the auditory pathway. An absent EABR in association with an abnormal stimulus artefact (identified by an integrity test) is suggestive of a malfunctioning electrode channel. A well-defined EABR waveform with a steep amplitude I/O function is thought to suggest good neuronal survival (Smith and Simmons, 1983; Hall, 1990; Abbas and Brown, 1993). The presence of these characteristics on the EABR is therefore desirable, but their absence is not an automatic indicator of poor performance by the

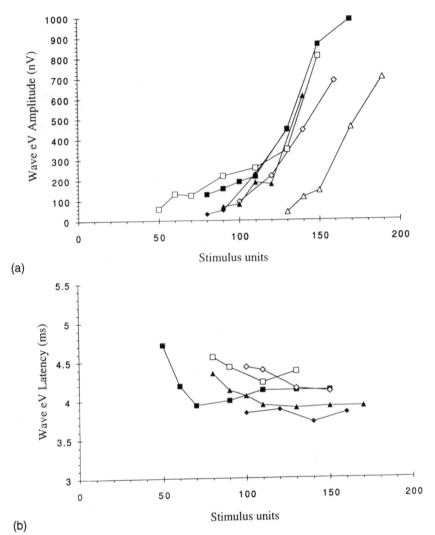

(a)

(b)

Figure 6.8 A selection of typical input/output (I/O) functions for (a) amplitude and (b) latency of the wave eV component of the EABR

implant user. Abbas and Brown (1991) were unable to demonstrate a significant correlation between the I/O function of the EABR and overall performance.

Electrically evoked stapedius reflex

The stapedius muscle reflex can be elicited electrically with a promontory or round window electrode, or through a specific channel of a cochlear implant. The reflex can be recorded using a conventional acoustic impedance meter, or detected by visual observation of movement of the muscle and tendon during implant surgery. The presence of a response confirms that the implant device is functioning. There are recent reports which suggest that the threshold of the electrically evoked stapedius reflex (ESRT) correlates with the comfort level of electrical stimulation experienced by patients (Battmer, Laszig and Lehnardt, 1990). The ESRT is therefore a potentially useful objective tool to check the functioning of the electrode array and to assist the fitting of a cochlear implant.

A typical electrical stimulus for measurement of the ESRT with the Nucleus cochlear implant is a 1-second burst of biphasic pulses with a pulse rate of 250 p.p.s. For analogue implant systems, such as the MED-EL device, a low frequency 1-second sine wave electrical stimulus can be used (Stephan, Welzl-Muller and Stiglbrunner, 1991). An acoustic impedance measurement of the reflex on the contralateral side to the implanted ear can be carried out either during or after surgery. A train of 5 or 10 stimulus bursts, with a repetition rate of around 1 second, should elicit a repeatable response. The repetitive stimulus will assist detection of the reflex. An alternative technique for measurement of the reflex is carried out during implant surgery. Movement and contraction of the stapedius muscle and tendon, evoked by a single 1-second stimulus burst, is observed through the operating microscope by the surgeon before closure of the middle ear (Sheppard et al., 1992). The stimulus intensity which just initiates the slightest movement is recorded as threshold of the response. Detection of this small movement often relies on observation of a slight change in the reflected light from the microscope, rather than observing the movement directly. Measurement of the ESRT during surgery can, however, be affected by the anaesthetic procedure. Muscle relaxants may inhibit the reflex, and nitrous oxide can influence measurements of the acoustic impedance on the contralateral side as a result of changes in middle-ear pressure. These anaesthetic regimes should be discontinued before measurement of the ESRT.

Most studies using the acoustic impedance technique have been conducted on adults, and the ESRT has been absent in a significant number of subjects: 24% (Battmer et al., 1990), 48% (Stephan, Welzl-Muller and Stiglbrunner, 1991). Explanations for the absence of the ESRT include inadequate current levels, insufficient number of surviving neurons, middle-ear pathology and lack of patient cooperation. The increased prevalence of middle-ear pathology in young children will add to the incidence of an absent reflex using the impedance method to measure the response. Absence of a reflex should therefore be interpreted with caution.

The incidence of an absent reflex, using visual observation of the stapedius during surgery to detect the response, is lower than for the impedance technique. A series of 14 children implanted with the Nucleus device have been studied using electrical stimulation in stimulus mode with a CG reference (Sheppard et al., 1992). In one of these patients the surgeon could not visualise the stapedius reliably. Of the remaining 13 children there were 121 threshold measurements carried out, of which 21 (17%) showed no reflex response at maximal stimulus level. Most of these no response conditions were recorded on the mid-range channels of the electrode array, and reflexes were still present on the apical and basal electrodes.

Integrity tests

Measurement of the electrical component of the stimulus artefact can be employed to check the integrity and functioning of individual channels of the electrode array. The amplitude and shape of the artefact produced by the stimulus can be characterised across different electrode channels and any malfunction in one or more channels will disturb this configuration. Methods of recording and analysis of the stimulus artefact have been termed the 'averaged electrode voltage' by Shallop (1993) and the 'stimulogram' by Almquist, Harris and Jonsson (1993). The artefact waveform can be recorded from surface scalp electrodes, similar to those used for the EABR, with signal averaging employed as necessary to improve the signal-to-noise amplitude ratio of the waveform. Several methodological factors affect the configuration of the artefact waveform including the site of the recording electrodes, the mode of presentation of the stimulus, the filter bandwidth of the signal amplifier, and whether there has been full insertion of the electrode array. An example of electrical stimulus artefact waveforms recorded from the EABR electrode sites in CG mode with a fully inserted Nucleus 22 channel electrode array are shown in Figure 6.9. These recordings demonstrate a progressive change in the amplitude and phase of the stimulus artefact from basal to apical electrode channels. Shallop (1993) recorded from electrodes on the ipsilateral and contralateral mastoids with bipolar stimulation and showed a different configuration, with amplitude of the artefact falling steadily from basal to apical electrode channels. Integrity testing is a useful objective way of checking the functioning of the implant and identifying possible electrode faults in young children where behavioural assessment may produce a confusing picture.

Prediction of electrical stimulation threshold

Intraoperative recording of the EABR during implant surgery is a popular protocol in young children. The threshold data can be used to predict the levels of electrical stimulation required for sensation of the

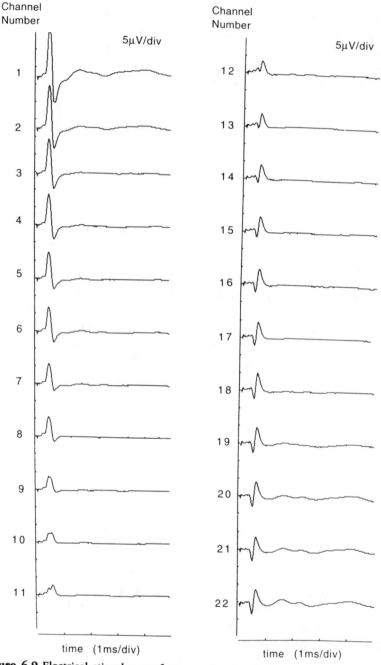

Figure 6.9 Electrical stimulus artefacts are shown which have been generated by pulse stimulation of individual electrode channels of the Nucleus electrode array. The biphasic pulse stimulus was presented in stimulus mode with an intensity of 150 stimulus units using a CG reference mode. The artefact signal was recorded from the EABR scalp electrodes with an amplifier filter bandwidth of 100 Hz to 3 kHz

stimulus during the initial fitting and tuning after implantation. The accuracy of this prediction is dependent on applying appropriate correction factors to the EABR threshold as demonstrated in a study using the Nucleus implant (Mason et al., 1993b). Analysis of the relationship between the intraoperative EABR threshold and the first reliable subjective threshold level (T level) obtained at around 4 weeks after surgery shows that the raw EABR threshold is on average less sensitive than the T level by about 35 stimulus units. Results from this study (81 thresholds in 24 children) are shown in Figures 6.10 and 6.11, and demonstrate the offset between the EABR threshold and T level, and spread in their relationship. This offset arises from the different pulse rates employed for each test (typically 31 p.p.s. for the EABR and 250 p.p.s. for the T level), the difficulties in the identification of a small EABR close-to-threshold, and possible change in the effective level of postoperative stimulation (Saudan et al., 1993). If a simple correction factor of 35 stimulus units is subtracted from all the EABR data, 80% of the corrected thresholds are within 30 stimulus units of the T level but only 58% are within 20 units. A similar offset between the EABR threshold and T level has been reported by Shallop et al. (1991).

A significant improvement in the prediction of the T level from the EABR is achieved when corrections for absolute intensity of stimulus threshold and channel number are taken into consideration (Mason et al., 1993b). Sensitivity of the EABR threshold is dependent on the absolute level of the stimulus threshold and is closer to T level for low intensity thresholds. The group mean values of EABR threshold and T level are both higher on the mid-range electrode channels (10 and 15) compared to channels 5 and 20, which is consistent with the 'bell-shaped' configuration normally observed in the common ground electrode configuration (Figure 6.10). There are 97.5% of corrected thresholds within 30 stimulus units of T level and 78% within 20 units when correction for absolute stimulus threshold and channel number is applied to the EABR threshold. The relative improvement in the relationship is evident by comparing the histograms shown in Figures 6.11 and 6.12. This improved level of accuracy in the relationship between the intraoperative EABR threshold and subsequent T level is extremely valuable during the initial fitting and tuning of the Nucleus cochlear implant in very young children.

Dynamic range

Threshold and comfort levels for electrical stimulation define the upper and lower limits of the dynamic range. An objective prediction of the dynamic range can be derived from the corrected EABR threshold and the ESRT. In patients with a wide dynamic range (typically 60 stimulus units in the Nucleus device), the clinical value of this prediction

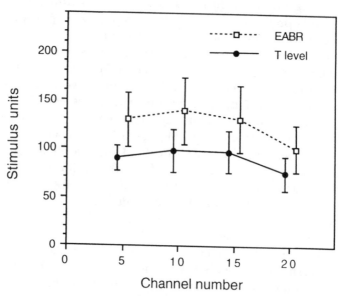

Figure 6.10 Group mean values (± 1 standard deviation) for the intraoperative EABR threshold and the first reliable subjective threshold (T level) for electrode channels 20, 15, 10 and 5 (from Mason et al., 1993b). The stimuli were presented via a Nucleus electrode array in stimulus mode with a CG reference mode

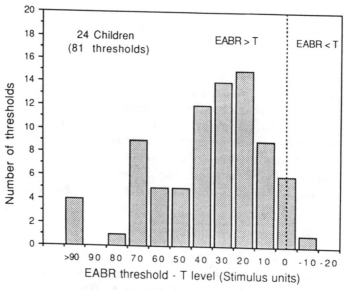

Figure 6.11 The typical distribution of the relationship between the raw intraoperative EABR threshold and the first reliable subjective threshold (T level). The mean offset between the two measurements is 35 stimulus units. (From Mason et al., 1993b)

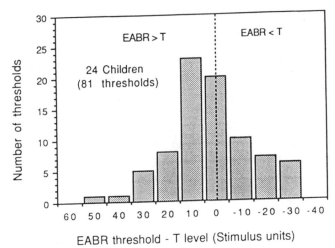

Figure 6.12 The distribution in the relationship between the EABR threshold and subsequent T level after correction for the absolute stimulus threshold and electrode channel number. There is clearly a marked improvement in their relationship when compared with the results presented in Figure 6.11

will be affected to a lesser extent by any inaccuracy in the EABR and ESRT measurements compared to patients with a very narrow dynamic range. Additional care must therefore be exercised in applying objective predictions when the difference between the corrected EABR threshold and ESRT is typically less than 30 stimulus units.

Pre-implant assessment

The suitability of a cochlear implant as a means of hearing rehabilitation depends on the availability of electrically excitable auditory neurons which will subsequently result in auditory sensation and perception. Presently there are no direct means to measure and quantify the level of this neuronal survival. An indirect approach is to make a preoperative assessment of whether electrical stimulation of the ear results in either auditory sensation or the generation of an EABR waveform.

Subjective stimulation tests

An electrical stimulus can be applied to the promontory in the middle ear using a trans-tympanic needle electrode and many patients will experience some degree of auditory sensation. In adults this test procedure is relatively straightforward and requires only a local anaesthetic. However, implementation of this electrode technique in older children is more difficult and is impossible in young children without general anaesthesia.

Electrical stimulation with a needle electrode positioned at the round window niche or a ball electrode on the round window is considered to be more sensitive than the promontory. However, placement of the electrode at the round window requires some visualisation of landmarks in the lateral cochlear wall via a small tympanotomy or tympano-meatal flap. Promontory stimulation is therefore a preferred first approach in adults, with round window stimulation reserved for those cases where the initial promontory test is negative. An absence of any acoustic sensation with these preoperative electrical tests may be a contraindication for cochlear implantation (Kileny et al., 1992b), although other workers (Gantz et al., 1993) report considerable variability in the ability of preoperative tests to predict audiological performance with multichannel cochlear implants.

Pre-implant electrically evoked auditory brain-stem response

In patients where a pre-implant assessment of a subjective response to promontory stimulation is not practicable, the EABR may offer the possibility of an alternative objective investigation. This technique is an attractive approach for young children below the age of 10 years. It has been suggested that the threshold and growth function (amplitude I/O function) of the EABR may have the ability to predict the extent of neuronal survival (Kileny, 1991; Shallop, 1993). The drawback regarding investigation of this procedure, is however, that a general anaesthetic is required for electrode placement in a young child. Some workers have also experienced difficulty in recording reliable and consistent EABR waveforms using extracochlear stimulation when compared with the intracochlear method (Kasper, Pelizzone and Montandon, 1991).

Evaluation of a child for implantation already involves a number of investigations which may require a general anaesthetic or at least sedation, such as ERA, radiology (high resolution computed tomography scan) or magnetic resonance imaging. The possibility of combining a pre-implant EABR assessment with other investigations under the same anaesthetic session should be investigated. A first step towards introduction and investigation of the pre-implant EABR into the evaluation protocol is described by Kilney et al. (1992a). In this study recordings of the EABR are carried out immediately before implant surgery after the child has been anaesthetised. The ear which gives the most sensitive EABR threshold and the steepest growth function is then selected for implantation, providing that there are no other contraindications which have to be taken into consideration such as ossification of the cochlea.

Future developments

Electrophysiological investigation of patients in both the preoperative and postoperative periods of cochlear implantation is still at an early stage of development. In the next few years we should see a better understanding and improved application of potentials evoked by electrical stimulation. This applies not only to the EABR but also to other responses such as the MMN and the P300 cognitive potentials. The characteristics of these responses are likely to be dependent on the type of implant device and the mode of stimulation. These differences should become more clearly defined as the number of investigations and published reports from different implant centres increases.

The value of objective electrophysiological tests in the expanding field of cochlear implantation in young children is now well recognised, and considerable time and effort are likely to be devoted to this work. In particular the potential use of the EABR as an objective preoperative indicator of neuronal survival, as an alternative to subjective promontory and round window stimulation tests, is an ongoing area of development. The immediate future should also see the relationships between the EABR and subjective stimulation thresholds, and the stapedius reflex thresholds and comfort levels, becoming more clearly defined. The techniques employed for stimulation and data collection are likely to experience future change and development in order to optimise and improve our understanding of test data. This is the beginning of a new era in the electrophysiological investigation of auditory function in young children and we should look forward to an exciting and rewarding future.

References

Abbas, P.J. (1988). Electrophysiology of the auditory system. *Clinical Physics and Physiological Measurement,* **9**, 1–31.

Abbas, P.J. and Brown, C.J. (1991). Electrically evoked auditory brainstem response: Growth of response with current level. *Hearing Research,* **51**, 123–138.

Abbas, P.J. and Brown, C.J. (1993). Comparison of EAP, EABR and psychophysical data from human cochlear implant users: Level effects. Presented at the 3rd International Cochlear Implant Conference, Innsbruck, April 4–7 1993.

Abramovich, S. (1990). *Electric Response Audiometry in Clinical Practice.* Edinburgh: Churchill Livingstone.

Achor, L.J. and Starr, A. (1980). Auditory brainstem responses in the cat. I. Intracranial and extracranial recordings. *Electroencephalography and Clinical Neurophysiology,* **48**, 154–173.

Allum, J.H.J., Shallop, J.K., Hotz, M. and Pfaltz, C.R. (1990). Characteristics of electrically evoked 'auditory' brainstem responses elicited with the Nucleus 22-electrode intracochlear implant. *Scandinavian Audiology,* **19**, 263–267.

Almqvist, B., Harris, H. and Jonsson, K-E. (1993). The stimulogram. Presented at the 3rd International Cochlear Implant Conference, Innsbruck, Austria, 4–7 April 1993.

Battmer, R-D., Laszig, R. and Lehnhardt, E. (1990). Electrically elicited stapedius reflex in cochlear implant patients. *Ear and Hearing,* **11**, 370–374.

Berger, H. (1929), (1930). On the electroencephalogram of man. In P. Gloor (ed.), *Hans Berger on the Electroencephalogram of Man, Electroencephalography and Clinical Neurophysiology*, Suppl. 28, 37. Amsterdam: Elsevier, 1969.

Brix, R. and Gedlicka, W. (1991). Late cortical auditory potentials evoked by electrostimulation in deaf and cochlear implant patients. *European Archives of Oto-Rhino-Laryngology*, **248**, 442–444.

Brown, C.J. and Abbas, P.J. (1990). Electrically evoked whole-nerve action potentials: Data from human cochlear implant users. *Journal of the Acoustical Society of America*, **88**, 1385–1391.

Davis. H. (1976). Brainstem and other responses in electrical response audiometry. *Annals of Otology*, **85**, 3–14.

Davis, H., Davis, P.A., Loomis, A.L., Harvey, E.N. and Hobart, G. (1939). Electrical reactions of the human brain to auditory stimulation during sleep. *Journal of Neurophysiology*, **2**, 500–514.

Davis, H. and Hirsh, S.K. (1979). A slow brainstem response for low-frequency audiometry. *Audiology*, **18**, 445–461.

Davis, P.A. (1939). Effects of acoustic stimuli on the waking human brain. *Journal of Neurophysiology*, **2**, 494–499.

Djourno, A. and Eyries, C (1957). Prosthese auditive par excitation electrique a distance du nerf sensoriel a l'aide d'un bobinage inclus a demeure. *Presse Medicale*, **35**, 14–17.

Drift, van der J.F.C., Brocaar, M.P. and van Zanten, G.A. (1987). The relation between the pure tone audiogram and the click auditory brainstem response threshold in cochlear hearing loss. *Audiology*, **26**, 1–10.

Finitzo-Hieber, T. and Friel-Patti, S. (1985). Conductive hearing loss and the ABR. In J.T. Jacobson (ed.), *The Auditory Brainstem Response*, pp. 113–132. San Diego, CA: College-Hill Press.

Game, C.J.A., Thomson, D.R. and Gibson, W.P.R. (1990). Measurement of auditory brainstem responses evoked by electrical stimulation with a cochlear implant. *British Journal of Audiology*, **24**, 145–149.

Gantz, B.J., Woodworth, G.G., Knutson, J.F., Abbas, P.J. and Tyler, R.S. (1993). Multivariate predictors of success with cochlear implants. *Advances in Oto-Rhino-Laryngology*, **48**, 153–167.

Gibbin, K.P. (1992). Paediatric cochlear implantation. *Archives of Disease in Childhood*, **67**, 669–671.

Gibson, W.P.R. (1978). *Essentials of Clinical Electric Response Audiometry*. London: Churchill Livingstone.

Gray, R.F. and Baguley, D.M. (1990). Electrical stimulation of the round window: A selection procedure for single-channel cochlear implantation. *Clinical Otolaryngology*, **15**, 29–34.

Gyo, K. and Yanagihara, N. (1980). Electrically and acoustically evoked brainstem responses in guinea pig. *Acta Oto-Laryngologica (Stockholm)*, **90**, 25–31.

Hall, R.D. (1990). Electrically evoked auditory brainstem responses (EABR) provide good estimates of surviving spiral ganglion cells in deaf rats. Abstract of paper presented at the Association for Research in Otolaryngology, St Petersburg Beach, Florida, February 4–8 1990.

Hashimoto, I. (1982). Auditory evoked potentials from the human midbrain: Slow brain stem responses. *Electroencephalography and Clinical Neurophysiology*, **53**, 652–657.

House, W.F. (1991). Cochlear implants in children: past and present perspectives. *American Journal of Otology*, 12 (Suppl.), 1–2.

Jacobson, J.T. (1985). *The Auditory Brainstem Response*. San Diego, CA: College-Hill Press.

Jewett, D.L. and Williston, J.S. (1971). Auditory-evoked far fields averaged from the scalp of humans. *Brain*, **94**, 681–696.

Kasper, A., Pelizzone, M. and Montandon, P. (1991). Intracochlear potential distribution with intracochlear and extracochlear electrical stimulation in humans. *Annals of Otology, Rhinology and Laryngology*, **100**, 812–816.

Kileny, P.R. (1991). Use of electrophysiologic measures in the management of children with cochlear implants: Brainstem, middle latency, and cognitive (P300) responses. *American Journal of Otology* (Suppl.),**12**, 37–42.

Kileny, P., Kemink, J.L. and Miller, J.M. (1989). An intrasubject comparison of electric and acoustic middle latency responses. *American Journal of Otology*, **10**, 23–27.

Kileny, P.R., Zimmerman-Phillips, S., Zwolan, T., Lougheed, L. and Kemink, J. (1992a). Preoperative EABR in paediatric cochlear implant candidates: classification and follow-up. Presented at the First European Symposium on Paediatric Cochlear Implantation, Nottingham, September 1992.

Kileny, P.R., Zwolan, T., Zimmerman-Phillips, S. and Kemink, J. (1992b). A comparison of round-window and transtympanic promontory electric stimulation in cochlear implant candidates. *Ear and Hearing*, **13**, 294–299.

Kraus, N., McGee, T., Sharma, A., Carrell, T. and Nicol, T. (1992). Mismatch negativity event-related potential elicited by speech stimuli. *Ear and Hearing*, **13**, 158–164.

Kraus, N., Micco, A.G., Koch, D.B., McGee, T., Carrell, T., Sharma, A., Wiet, R.J. and Weingarten, C.Z. (1993). The mismatch negativity cortical evoked potential elicited by speech in cochlear implant users. *Hearing Research*, **65**, 118–124.

Lightfoot, G.R. and Mason, S.M. (1993). Electric response audiometry (ERA): principles, techniques and clinical applications. Course notes from the Liverpool ERA Course, University of Liverpool and Royal Liverpool Hospital.

McCormick, B. (1991). Paediatric cochlear implantation in the United Kingdom – a delayed journey on a well marked route. *British Journal of Audiology*, **25**, 145–149.

McCormick, B., Gibbin, K.P., Lutman, M.E. and O'Donoghue, G.M. (1993). Late partial recovery from meningitis deafness after cochlear implantation: a case study. *American Journal of Otology*, **14**, 1–3.

Mahoney, T. M. (1985). Auditory brainstem response hearing aid applications. In J.T. Jacobson (ed.), *The Auditory Brainstem Response*, pp. 349–370. San Diego, CA: College-Hill Press.

Mason, S.M. (1984). Effects of high-pass filtering on the detection of the auditory brainstem response. *British Journal of Audiology*, **18**, 155–161.

Mason, S.M. (1993). Electric response audiometry. In B. McCormick (ed.), *Paediatric Audiology, 0–5 Years*, 2nd edn pp. 187–249. London: Whurr.

Mason, S.M., McCormick, B. and Wood, S. (1988). Auditory brainstem response in paediatric audiology. *Archives of Disease in Childhood*, **63**, 465–467.

Mason, S.M., Singh, C.B. and Brown, P.M. (1980). Assessment of non-invasive electrocochleography. *Journal of Laryngology and Otology*, **94**, 707–718.

Mason, S.M., Sheppard S., Garnham, C.W., Lutman, M.E., O'Donoghue, G.M. and Gibbin, K.P. (1993a). Application of intraoperative recordings of electrically evoked ABRs in a paediatric cochlear implant programme. *Advances in Oto-Rhino-Laryngology*, **48**, 136–141.

Mason, S.M., Sheppard S., Garnham, C.W., Lutman, M.E., O'Donoghue, G.M. and Gibbin, K.P. (1993b). Improving the relationship of intraoperative EABR threshold to T-level in young children receiving the Nucleus cochlear implant. *Proceedings of the 3rd International Cochlear Implant Conference*, Innsbruck, April 4–7 1993 (in press).

Meikle, M. B., Gillette, R.G. and Godfrey, F.A. (1977). Comparison of electrically and acoustically evoked responses in the auditory cortex of the guinea pig: Implications for a cochlear prosthesis. *Transactions of the American Academy of Ophthalmology and Otology*, 84, 183–192.

Millard, R.E., McAnally, K.I. and Clark, G.M. (1992). A gated differential amplifier for recording physiological responses to electrical stimulation. *Journal of Neuroscience Methods*, 44, 81–84.

Miyamoto, R.T. (1986). Electrically evoked potentials in cochlear implants. *The Laryngoscope*, 96, 178–185.

Miyamoto, R.T. and Osberger, M.J. (1991). Cochlear implants in children. *The American Journal of Otology* (Suppl.), 12.

Mokatoff, B., Schulman-Galambos, C. and Galambos, R. (1977). Brain stem auditory evoked response in children. *Archives of Otolaryngology*, 103, 38–43.

Moller, A.R. and Jannetta, P.J. (1984). Neural generators of the brainstem auditory evoked potential. In R.H. Nodar and C. Barber (eds), *Evoked Potentials II*, pp. 137–144. Boston: Butterworth.

Muller-Deile, J., Schmidt, B.J. and Rudert, H. (1993). Facial stimulation – a problem in speech processor programming. Presented at the 3rd International Cochlear Implant Conference, Innsbruck, April 4–7 1993.

O'Donoghue, G.M. (1992). Cochlear implants in children. *Journal of the Royal Society of Medicine*, 85, 655–658.

Odenthal, D.W. and Eggermont, J.J. (1974). Clinical electrocochleography. *Acta Oto-Laryngologica Supplementum*, 316, 62–74.

Oviatt, D.L. and Kileny, P.R. (1991). Auditory event-related potentials elicited from cochlear implant recipients and hearing subjects. *American Journal of Audiology*, 1, 48–55.

Pelizzone, M., Kasper, K. and Montandon, P. (1989). Electrically evoked responses in cochlear implant patients. *Audiology*, 28, 230–238.

Picton, T.W., Hillyard, S.A., Krausz, H.I. and Galambos, R. (1974). Human auditory evoked potentials. I. Evaluation of components. *Electroencephalography and Clinical Neurophysiology*, 36, 179–190.

Picton, T.W., Champagne, S.C. and Kellett, A.J.C. (1992). Human auditory evoked potentials recorded using maximum length sequences. *Electroencephalography and Clinical Neurophysiology*, 84, 90–100.

Portmann, M., Lebert, G. and Aran J.-M. (1967). Potentiels cochleares obtenus chez l'homme en dehors de toute intervention chirurgicale. *Revue de Laryngologie*, 88, 157–164.

Regan, D. (1989). Cognitive processes and motor action. In D. Regan (ed.), *Human Brain Electrophysiology*, pp. 210–250. New York: Elsevier Science.

Saudan, O., Pelizzone, M. and Montandon, P. (1993). Peroperative and postoperative recordings of electrically evoked auditory brainstem responses (EABR) in totally deaf patients. Presented at the 3rd International Cochlear Implant Conference, Innsbruck, April 4–7 1993.

Schwartz, D.M. and Berry, G.A. (1985). Normative aspects of the ABR. In J.T. Jacobson (ed.), *The Auditory Brainstem Response*, p. 83. San Diego, CA: College-Hill Press.

Shallop, J.K. (1993). Objective electrophysiological measures from cochlear implant patients. *Ear and Hearing*, 14, 58–63.

Shallop, J.K., Beiter, A.L., Goin, D.W. and Mischke, R.E. (1990). Electrically evoked auditory brainstem response (EABR) and middle latency responses (EMLR) obtained from patients with the Nucleus multichannel cochlear implant. *Ear and Hearing*, **11**, 5–15.

Shallop, J.K., VanDyke, L., Goin, D.W. and Mischke, R.E. (1991). Prediction of behavioural threshold and comfort values for Nucleus 22-channel implant patients from electrical auditory brain stem response test results. *Annals of Otology, Rhinology and Laryngology*, **100**, 896–898.

Sheppard, S., Mason, S.M., Lutman, M.E., Gibbin, K.P. and O'Donoghue, G.M. (1992). Intraoperative electrical stapedial reflex measurements in young children receiving cochlear implants. Presented at the First European Symposium on Paediatric Cochlear Implantation, Nottingham, September 1992.

Smith, L. and Simmons, F.B. (1983). Estimating eighth nerve survival by electrical stimulation. *Annals of Otology, Rhinology and Laryngology*, **92**, 19–25.

Sohmer, H. and Feinmesser, M. (1967). Cochlear action potentials recorded from the external ear in man. *Annals of Otology, Rhinology and Laryngology*, **76**, 427–435.

Staller, S.J. (1991). Multichannel cochlear implants in children. *Ear and Hearing* (Suppl.), **12**.

Stapells, D.R., Picton, T.W., Perez-Abalo, M., Read, D. and Smith, A. (1985). Frequency specificity in evoked potential audiometry. In J.T. Jacobson (ed.), *The Auditory Brainstem Response*, pp. 147–180., San Diego, College-Hill Press.

Stapells, D.R., Galambos, R., Costello, J.A. and Makeig, S. (1988). Inconsistency of auditory middle latency and steady-state responses in infants. *Electroencephalography and Clinical Neurophysiology*, **71**, 289–295.

Starr, A. and Brackmann, D.E. (1979). Brainstem potentials evoked by electrical stimulation of the cochlea in human subjects. *Annals of Otology, Rhinology and Laryngology*, **88**, 550–556.

Stephan, K., Welzl-Muller, K. and Stiglbrunner H. (1991). Acoustic reflex in patients with cochlear implants (analog stimulation). *American Journal of Otology*, **12**, 48–51.

Stockard, J.J. and Rossiter, M.A. (1977). Clinical and pathologic correlates of brain stem auditory response abnormalities. *Neurology*, **27**, 316–325.

Taylor, M.J. (1991). EPs and ERPs in paediatrics. In C. Barber and M. Taylor (eds), *Evoked Potentials Review*, No. 4, pp. 1–14. Nottingham: IEPS Publications.

Thornton, A.R.D. (1987). Electrophysiological measures of hearing function in hearing disorders. *British Medical Bulletin*, **43**, 92–939.

Chapter 7
Fitting and programming the external system

SARAH SHEPPARD

For any cochlear implant system to function, external equipment is required which delivers power and the appropriately modified signal to the implanted electrode array. The external components are the microphone, the speech processor and the transcutaneous transmitter or the percutaneous plug which communicate the signal to the implanted electrodes. These components must be connected together and fitted to the patient (Figure 7.1). Additionally the speech processor must be appropriately set so that a signal, which is perceived as audible but not uncomfortable to the patient, is delivered to the electrode array. To set the processor up properly measurements have to be made individually for each patient. For single-channel analogue systems, this requires measurement of the minimal audible level (the threshold) and the maximum comfortable level of loudness for frequencies across the approximate range of 60 Hz to 4 kHz (Hochmair-Desoyer, 1986). For multichannel systems thresholds and maximum comfortable levels of loudness, sometimes known as the comfort level, are measured for each active electrode channel (Parkin and Stewart, 1988; Beiter, Staller and Dowell, 1991). This is the assessment of the dynamic range of electrical stimulation for each patient. The dynamic range is the range between the thresholds and the maximum comfortable levels, and is affected by several factors such as the characteristics of the stimulus, electrode configuration and placement, and physiological factors of neural density and distribution. The dynamic range for electrical stimulation is, however, narrow, being equivalent to less than 15–20 dB, (Pfingst, Spelman and Sutton, 1980; Patrick et al., 1990). Different cochlear implant systems use different units to express the dynamic range but all relate to the current density. Sometimes arbitrary number values are used; other systems use units of current or electrical decibels. The processor has to be programmed to deliver all the signal information into the narrow physiological dynamic range of each

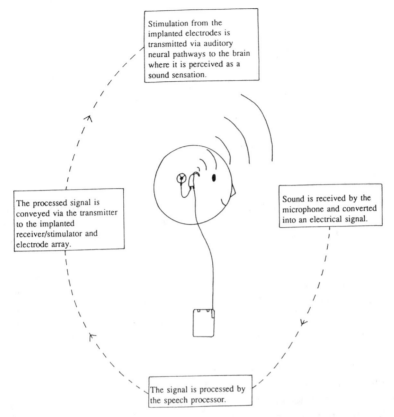

Figure 7.1 Diagrammatic representation of how the different components of a cochlear implant system function to induce a sensation of hearing

patient where the signal will be heard comfortably. If the dynamic range is set too wide, or too high, signals may be above maximum comfortable level and will be painful; if it is set too low signals may be below the minimum audible level and will not be heard. If the dynamic range is set too narrowly, the subject will be less able to distinguish different loudness levels (Figure 7.2). The measurement of dynamic range is the main goal in the fitting and programming of any cochlear implant system and is the basis of setting initial stimulation parameters for the processor. Further measurements are required with different implant systems to fine tune the signal sent to the implanted electrodes.

Clinic and equipment for device fitting and programming

All cochlear implant systems require specialist equipment for programming speech processors. Most systems use personal computers with

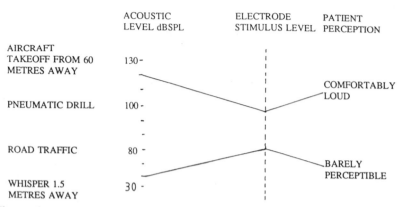

Figure 7.2 Diagram showing the need for signal compression to allow the broad acoustic dynamic range to be represented as fully as possible, within the narrow electrical dynamic range available for comfortable stimulation with a cochlear implant

device-specific interface cards fitted to them. Many systems also have a separate interface unit which is connected to the computer. Stimulus parameters are set by the computer keyboard and sometimes also by hand-held stimulus attenuators. The interface unit delivers signals to the patient via a test coil or transmitter and lead, which may or may not be connected via a speech processor depending on the system used. The electrical safety of the stimulating source should be verified by qualified electronics personnnel. It may be necessary to use an isolation transformer in some cases, because during testing there is a direct connection between the patient and the mains electricity. For the programming of cochlear implant systems to be carried out optimally with young children, the audiological staff should be experienced with audiological test techniques for young hearing-impaired children under the age of 5 years. Additional training in the use of electrical stimulation with reference to cochlear implants will be required. The American Speech–Language–Hearing Association (1992) have laid down guidelines for audiologists working with cochlear implant patients; these have the aim of ensuring the quality of care, welfare, safety and comfort of patients for practitioners.

Two testers are usually employed to program the speech processors of young children; one operates the programming equipment while the other is free to work with the child, encouraging and rewarding appropriately. Young children may respond in a variety of very subtle ways particularly during initial stimulation. It is therefore advantageous to have two people observing the child, one of whom can give full attention to the child. Young children may be distracted or distressed by a lot of high technology equipment; for this reason in the author's programme the cochlear implant programming equipment may be operated from an observation room adjacent to the clinic (Figure 7.3). The use of the observation room also ensures that any response or change in behaviour is the result of an auditory stimulus via the implant and not of any visual clue from testers, parents or other observers. Severely and profoundly deaf children are often more aware of visual clues than normally hearing children.

Programming training

Before introducing and fitting the speech processor and headset, it is helpful to give the implanted child some indication of the process of programming the cochlear implant system. If dummy equipment is available the child can be allowed to see, handle and wear the dummy equipment before initial stimulation. This will minimise any apprehension about new equipment. Older children may have sufficient language for this information to be communicated by sign or written language, but most young children's language will be inadequate. It is, however, possible to convey some basic information by using colouring books which give a simple pictorial explanation of the process (see Chapter 3). Some children may be helped by observing another child or an adult during a programming session before initial programming, to reduce any stress or negative feelings experienced by the child during this period.

During the pre-implant assessment process the child will have

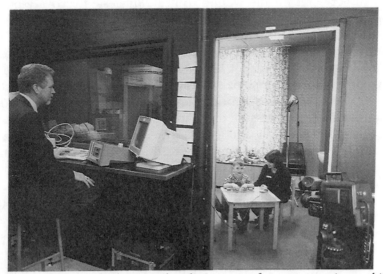

Figure 7.3 Photograph showing the clinic set-up for programming a child's cochlear implant. One tester works in the clinic with full attention devoted to the child while the second tester operates the programming equipment in the observation room

undergone extensive audiological testing. This will probably have included testing where the child is conditioned to respond to a stimulus that may be auditory, visual or vibrotactile (see Chapter 4). The child should therefore already be capable of, and experienced in, some of the test techniques required to program the speech processor. Some clinicians advocate pre-programming training, using visual and vibrotactile stimuli with the child before initial stimulation (Mecklenburg et al., 1990; Beiter, Staller and Dowell, 1991). Distinctions such as on/off are relatively easy for young children to understand, but concepts such as quiet/loud and same/different will be more difficult, if not impossible, for recently implanted children under the age of 5 years. The benefit of pre-programming training also needs to be balanced against the tasks becoming boring for the child. Further conditioning and training should be reinforced during and after initial stimulation because the signal received through the implant will be different from anything previously experienced by the child. With experience of the hearing sensation afforded by the implant, children are then able to demonstrate understanding, such as loud versus quiet, same versus different and long versus short duration of sound stimuli.

Initial stimulation

Between 3 and 6 weeks after the operation, in which the internal part of the device is surgically implanted, the external part of the device can be fitted. Sufficient time must be allowed for the patient to recover from surgery and for the wound to heal. Suggested recovery periods for different implant systems vary (Roberts, 1991). This period of waiting can be difficult for parents but intraoperative test results give reassurance that there has been some auditory response recorded through the implant (see Chapter 6). Before starting the initial stimulation session, parents and professionals working with the child and, if appropriate, the child, should be informed about the programming procedure. There should be no pressure to complete a certain amount of measurements in the first session and it should be clear that this will be the first of many programming sessions before the processor is set optimally. Some children find their first experience of electrical stimulation of the cochlea very strange and appear to be unable to carry out test procedures which they have previously learned using visual or vibrotactile stimuli. It may be impossible to do more than just observe some children for any signs of response to stimulation during the initial session. It is important to reiterate to parents, teachers and other observers that immediate responses to sound by the child may not be evident and should not be forced during this period. If the child is able to understand, it is helpful to again inform him or her that sound through the implant will be different to what has been heard before, but with time, further programming and extensive rehabilitation, the sound should become more familiar and the child will be able to make more use of the sound sensation received through the implant.

Measurements of electrical stapedial reflex thresholds (ESRT) (Battmer, Laszig and Lehnhardt, 1990; Stephan, Welzl-Muller and Stiglbrumer, 1991) and electrically evoked auditory brain-stem responses (EABR) (Shallop et al., 1990, 1991; Mason et al., 1994) are helpful during initial stimulation. ESRT measurements are usually obtained for about 10 channels of the Nucleus 22 cochlear implant in the author's own program. These give an indication that individual electrode channels can elicit an auditory response but are at much higher stimulation levels than the child will tolerate initially. The upper limits of the dynamic range are therefore set well below the level of the ESRT for each electrode channel. EABR measurements are more directly useful because it is possible to obtain some indication of behavioural thresholds for electrode channels using the Nucleus device. The EABR thresholds are usually less sensitive than the behavioural threshold (T) levels with the Nucleus device. There is some variation between patients but, if analysed channel by channel, a high percentage of the EABR levels are less sensitive, although within 30 units of behavioural T levels (Mason et al., 1994). EABR and ESRT measurements have been discussed in more detail in Chapter 6. It is, therefore, possible to begin conditioning the child to a definite stimulus through the implant knowing that the level presented will not be uncomfortable. Threshold measurements can then be carried out on as many electrode channels as possible, with the Nucleus device, or at different frequencies for analogue-frequency-equalised single or multichannel devices.

Behavioural threshold measurements

Initially the dynamic range tolerated by the new implantee will be small but there is a wide range in sensitivity to electrical stimulation between different individuals. Patients are therefore tested individually, starting at a low level and ascending, until there is a response. If no intraoperative measures have been carried out it will be necessary to start at the lowest unit of stimulation to avoid over-stimulation. When EABR measurements have been obtained it may be possible to predict the region where stimulation will occur near the threshold, although the EABR is usually less sensitive than behavioural threshold levels. The closeness of EABR measurements to threshold measurements is influenced by the recording parameters used (Shallop et al., 1991; Mason et al., 1994). The child is encouraged to carry out a play activity such as putting a man in a boat or a peg in a board when they hear a sound. It may be necessary to obtain several clear responses at the same level, thus reinforcing conditioning of the child, before reducing the current to find the threshold. Once the child stops responding the current level is raised again to find the lowest level at which the child consistently responds – this is the threshold. The use of clear on/off signals rather than a gradually increasing pulse train facilitates the measurement of thresholds. This type of conditioning task is the same as that used widely in paediatric audiology for performance testing (McCormick, 1988) and play audiometry (Wood, 1988). If young children find the first stimulation session overwhelming or distressing and are not able to carry out conditioning tasks, it may be possible to obtain some idea of where the threshold is by observing changes in the child's behaviour. Examples of behaviour changes with stimulation are stilling, questioning, adverse responses, touching the implanted side of the head or the test coil, or changes in facial expression. These responses do, however, habituate fairly quickly and some children show no apparent response at all. Young children will also show a similar range of behaviours if the sound stimulus is too loud or uncomfortable and such responses should be interpreted with caution. For this reason intraoperative EABR measurements are very valuable. If the recording parameters are such that behavioural thresholds can be estimated from EABR thresholds, these can form the basis of the first conservative processor settings for a small number of electrodes for children where behavioural testing of thresholds is not possible during the first session.

Behavioural maximum comfortable loudness level assessment

Having obtained at least some measurements of thresholds, it is necessary to set the upper level of the dynamic range. It is very important that cochlear implant systems are set so that stimulation is audible but also comfortable. If the maximum comfortable level is exceeded the child may become anxious because the sensation may be unpleasant, and is likely to be reluctant to use the speech processor or to reject it completely. With all implant systems it is usual practice to begin at a low level of stimulation, just above the threshold, and gradually to increase the level of the stimulus while the patient gives some indication of how loud the sound is becoming. For analogue multichannel devices the gain is adjusted gradually on each channel (Parkin and Stewart, 1988). For single-channel broad-band analogue devices, signals of different frequencies are presented to the patient who then gives an indication of loudness level. When measurements have been made across the frequency range, the frequency response of the speech processor is adjusted accordingly (Hochmair-Desoyer, 1986). With the Nucleus implant, which is a multichannel pulsatile device, a maximum comfortable level or comfort (C) level must be found separately for each channel because there are variations in C levels for different channels; some children, usually from the age of 7 years or older, may be able to indicate when a sound is quiet, loud or too loud as the level of stimulation is increased (Mac-Pherson et al., 1991).

Graduated written scales from quiet to too loud may be used for older children who can read well. These may be simplified down to three steps – quiet, loud, too loud – or two steps – okay, stop. Children often recognise a green light as meaning 'go' or continue stimulation and a red light for stop. Pictures designed to represent loudness growth have been used with children such as faces with changing expressions (Staller, Beiter and Brimacombe, 1991). Sometimes it may, however, be difficult to determine whether the child has understood the concept as intended. Some children will just point to the picture they find most amusing and others may just gradually move from one to another without regard to the loudness levels. For all of these approaches to determining maximum comfortable loudness, children will need practice and guidance before reliable results can be obtained. Children aged under 7 years and a significant proportion of older children will not be able to carry out this sort of distinction in the early stages of stimulation. Children generally need some experience with using their implants before they are able to distinguish loud and quiet. For this reason it is necessary to observe the child while gradually increasing the stimulus level until a small dynamic range is obtained at each frequency (analogue system) or electrode (pulsatile, multichannel system). With the Nucleus device, single electrode maps can be created and the upper limit of the dynamic range of an individual channel can be gradually increased while talking to the child and playing with noisy toys and musical instruments. This has the advantage that the child has some control of the sound making and the sound stimulus is more 'realistic', unlike a gradually increasing series of bursts of pulses (Mecklenburg et al., 1990). The clinician must be vigilant in looking for any adverse responses, such as obvious distress, but also stilling, touching the test coil or the side of the face, quietness, change in facial expression or facial twitching. Any of these signs are indications of the loudness discomfort level which is above the most comfortable level where C levels should be set. During initial stimulation it is advisable to set a small and therefore conservative dynamic range, even if there is no apparent discomfort, because it is unpleasant for the child even to approach an uncomfortable level of stimulation on several channels at this early stage. A stronger reaction is also normally observed when all channels are activated together even if very little reaction was seen to individual stimulation of channels. At the first stimulation the aim is to give the child some experience of stimulation through the implant that is pleasant and comfortable. With this experience the child's responses will be more definitive at subsequent sessions thus facilitating further tuning of the system.

Programming or setting of the speech processor

Once some threshold and maximum comfort levels have been obtained, the speech processor can be set or programmed with the initial dynamic range for stimulation. For some devices settings on the speech processors are adjusted manually, whereas with others the processor has a microchip that is programmed from the computer and device interface. The Nucleus implant system is of the latter type and the programmed parameters in the speech processor are commonly referred to as the MAP. Some devices do not use all channels, but measurements are made on all available electrodes so that those with the best dynamic range can be selected for stimulation (Burian, Hochmair-Desoyer and Eisenwort, 1986; Parkin and Stewart, 1988). Less variation is generally found between individuals for measurement of threshold and maximum comfortable levels with analogue systems. With the MED-EL single-channel system a normalised frequency response has been derived from the thresholds and fitting curves of postlingually deafened adult patients. The normalised curve can be used with a minimum of one threshold measurement carried out with the child to obtain the initial processor settings (Kerber, Herka and Klasek, 1993). The child may show a variety of reactions to sound stimulation when first using the processor; if adverse reactions are seen it will be necessary to reduce the upper limit of the dynamic range or the number of electrodes activated. It is important to look for any sign of discomfort before the child leaves the clinic, using loud noisemakers over the operating range of frequencies for the implant system as a further check that the processor has not been set too loud. Children enjoy associating sound with objects and experimenting with musical instruments, and the noises of everyday objects or events can help the child have a positive first experience of sound through the implant system. For this reason it is helpful to have alternating programming and rehabilitation sessions to encourage the child to use the speech processor and start to associate sounds with their sources. Using the Nucleus device in a series of 32 children, 3–20 channels have been programmed in the first session with under 5 year olds and between 4 and 22 channels programmed for children over 5 years (Sheppard, Cope and Twomey, 1993). Staller, Beiter and Brimacombe (1991) report similar figures with a mean of 7.3 channels programmed on day 1 of stimulation for 2–5 year olds.

Follow-up programming sessions

Follow-up programming sessions are necessary to check the functioning of the different external components of the implant system, to monitor the appropriateness of the programmed parameters, and to adjust the processor settings or MAP on the basis of new measurements of threshold and maximum comfortable loudness levels. Implantees become more tolerant of electrical stimulation when they have had some experience of using their devices. They are also able to carry out threshold, maximum comfortable loudness levels and other measurements more precisely. It is therefore not realistic to expect to reach final settings for the speech processor without follow-up programming sessions. With children the increase in the upper level of stimulation and dynamic range is best achieved by gradually increasing stimulation levels over several sessions. ESRT measurements may prove to give guidance with the Nucleus device, although those levels are not usually reached until the dynamic range has been increased on several occasions and precise data linking ESRT with maximum comfortable loudness levels for different implant systems have not been established

In addition to checking previous measurements and increasing the dynamic range, new electrode channels can be activated at follow-up sessions. Any electrodes which give little or no response or unusual responses may indicate an electrode fault or non-auditory stimulation. It is important for these electrodes to be identified and deactivated. Even after programming changes are complete, yearly reviews are advisable, particularly for children, to check for any slight changes in programming resulting from physiological changes and also to identify any electrode or equipment problems which may not have been reported by the child.

The use of computer games is being considered by some clinics to help make the tasks of programming more interesting for children and to keep their attention, thus maintaining the maximum possible accuracy and minimising programming time (Boothroyd et al., 1992). Various techniques may be employed for threshold measurements; these mainly involve the child using a mouse button and being rewarded by an image or animation on the computer monitor. Games for maximum comfortable level measurements are more difficult but computer images of different sized, but equally attractive, objects could be used to convey increasing 'size' or loudness. Ideally it would be good to incorporate a clear stop signal that the child could activate to prevent the signal getting any louder. Care would be needed in developing such a game so that pressing the stop button would not be so rewarding as to encourage the child to stop increasing the dynamic range too soon. This will no doubt be developed further.

Additional considerations for tuning implants

The Nucleus multichannel intracochlear cochlear implant is currently the device used most widely with children (Patrick and Clarke, 1991) for reasons discussed in Chapter 2: considerable adult data show good results and suggest better performance than single-channel implants

and extracochlear implants, transcutaneous transmission, good support and back-up pledged by manufacturers. This device is also one of
the more complex to program. Owing to the variation in threshold (T)
and comfort (C) levels between patients and electrodes, measurements
must be carried out on all active channels of which up to 22 may be
used. This necessitates a lot of testing. In addition to T and C level
measurements, it is recommended that further testing be carried out to
determine relative loudness growth on different channels which can be
achieved by electrode balancing. This is important to ensure that the
relative loudness of sound in the signal is represented as truly as possible via the implant. Also, some electrodes produce a sensation of
sound but very little loudness growth, which may only be revealed
through balancing or asking the patient to express the level of loudness
on an electrode as the stimulus is gradually increased. If an electrode is
not functioning optimally it is better to deactivate it. In addition pitch
ranking can be carried out to determine whether the implantee perceives an even range of pitch across the electrode array following the
tonotopic arrangement of the cochlea. These tests are described by
Roberts (1991) and Tye-Murray (1993), and involve comparing and
contrasting the loudness and pitch perceived when different electrodes
are stimulated. This is a difficult task for adult implantees and it is often
impossible for young children to give meaningful results because it is
difficult for them to separate changes in loudness and pitch. Checking
the pitch perception through different channels of the Nucleus device
is, however, advised wherever possible. Any electrodes that the patient
indicates sound very different should be deactivated. With extracochlear multichannel stimulation this type of testing is less predictable
because the position of different electrodes placed on the promontory
does not necessarily give an indication of which frequency area of the
cochlea will be stimulated (Hortman et al., 1989). Also it is possible
that intracochlear multichannel electrodes placed inside a malformed
cochlea may not follow the expected pitch sequence when stimulated.
    With young children it is not always possible to achieve the most
optimal tuning of a complex implant system. With increasing maturity
and experience with their implants, more sophisticated testing can be
attempted. Young children may give an indication that an electrode
sounds different during T and C level testing by not responding confi-
dently or by being puzzled or distressed. Threshold and maximum
comfort levels may reveal an electrode channel with a very small
dynamic range or T and C levels very different to adjacent channels. If
this occurs then it may be advisable to consider deactivating the electrodes because it may be an indication of poor function. Some of the
newer devices give much more programming choice, such as the Laura
device (Peeters, Offeciers and Marquet, 1990) and the Clarion device
which permits either compressed analogue or continuous interleaved

sampling (Schindler and Kessler, 1992); this may provide the audiologist with difficult decisions about which to use with children. New programming strategies for existing devices may also introduce extra complexities to the programming process. In spite of difficulties in programming complex cochlear implants for children, many show good responses with their implants (Osberger et al., 1991; Staller et al., 1991; Tyler, 1993). It has been suggested that neural plasticity in young children may allow them to adapt to any imbalance in the signal. Some children accept MAP changes more readily than others.

Further considerations for programming with the Nucleus device include deciding which coding strategy and which stimulus mode to select for measurements and for creating the MAP. The stimulus mode refers to the way in which the current is directed within the cochlea. A variety of bipolar stimulus modes can be selected in which the current flows between the active and a specific return electrode. In bipolar (BP) mode the next apical electrode is the reference, in bipolar + 1 (BP + 1) mode, the next but one apical electrode is the reference and in bipolar + 2 (BP + 2) the next but two electrode is the reference, etc. An additional stimulus mode, which is a quasibipolar mode called common ground mode, is usually the preferred initial programming mode for children. In common ground mode, the designated active electrode uses a common return or reference made up of all the remaining electrodes in the array (Figure 7.4). Damaged or faulty electrodes are generally thought to be easier to detect in common ground mode and should an electrode problem occur the patient is less likely to experience over-stimulation when that electrode is active, compared with any bipolar mode where there is the possibility of the patient experiencing an unpleasant or loud sensation. Theoretically, as current is more specifically directed, bipolar modes of stimulation should stimulate more discrete groups of neurons and therefore discrimination of different sounds is theoretically enhanced. In practice no significant difference has yet been demonstrated between different stimulus modes, with some adult patients preferring common ground mode and some preferring a bipolar mode of stimulation (George et al., 1993).

For some children, most clinics consider programming in one of the bipolar modes if either some electrodes are outside the cochlea or optimum C levels cannot be reached in common ground mode. If the insertion of the electrode array is incomplete in common ground mode, current is more likely to spread and stimulate tissues outside the cochlea via electrodes positioned there. This may result in unpleasant non-auditory sensations and may not be immediately evident but become so as the dynamic range is increased on channels just inside the cochlea. To give a better dynamic range on these electrodes and prevent current spread to tissue outside the cochlea, it will be necessary to change from common ground to a bipolar stimulation mode,

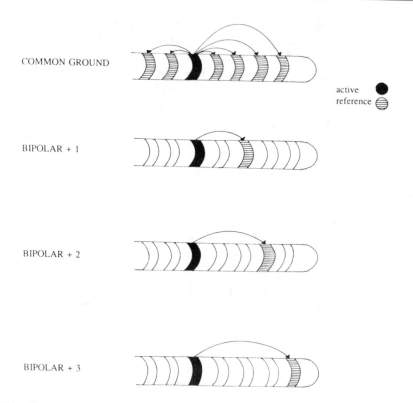

Figure 7.4 Diagram showing the different configurations of active and reference electrodes or stimulus modes, possible with the Nucleus cochlear implant

e.g. bipolar + 1, bipolar + 2, etc. Bipolar mode is rarely selected because the T and C levels are often too high. To change stimulus mode all the T and C levels have to be remeasured. Common ground mode of stimulation usually produces a bell-shaped MAP with larger dynamic ranges for electrodes in the middle part of the electrode array. For some patients it is not possible to reach a C level in common ground for electrodes in the middle of the array, and therefore loudness growth will not be even for different channels. If this 'topping out' situation arises, the reprogramming in one of the bipolar modes should be considered so that C levels can be set to give a more appropriate dynamic range.

Once all the measurements have been made, it is necessary to select a coding strategy for the Nucleus speech processor. The optimum coding strategy of the Nucleus device is currently Multipeak, where formant frequency peaks are extracted together with high-frequency filter band information (von Wallenberg and Battmer, 1991). This coding strategy is suitable for most patients except those with only a few electrodes inserted into the cochlea. One of a variety of simpler strategies needs to be considered because there may be too few channels for the Multipeak strategy to operate properly. If necessary, different frequency boundaries can be assigned to channels, e.g. with partial insertion of only a few channels (Balkany, Gantz and Nadol, 1988; Beiter, Staller and Dowell, 1991).

Length of time for programming with children

Considerable time is invested in programming speech processors for children both in terms of the number of hours of testing and also the time over which programming sessions are spread. Programming of the Nucleus implant is likely to be the most time-consuming because of the complexity of the device. As an indication of the time involved, it is interesting to look at the number of channels programmed in the first session and the timespan beyond which only minor changes in mapping are required. In a group of 19 children implanted below the age of 5 years, four had up to four channels programmed initially, five had 5–9 channels programmed, five had 10–14 channels programmed and seven had 15–20 channels programmed. In a group of children aged between 5 and 12 years at implantation, only one had less than four channels programmed initially, nine had 10–20 channels programmed initially and three had more than 20 channels programmed. An average of 21 hours, over a period of up to 8 months, is required to programme all active channels. Over 27 hours has been required to reach a final MAP in this group of under 5 year olds, whereas children older than 5 years required between 18 and 37 hours of tuning sessions spread over 2 years. This represents considerably more time than, for example, for fitting and checking hearing aids or programming implants for adults. Different clinics offer different arrangements for programming which will depend on the flexibility of clinic staff, age of patients and how far the families of implanted children live from the clinic. If the clinic is flexible enough to be able to offer many appointments at an early stage, this may help to programme processors more quickly, but time between appointments is needed for the child to adapt gradually to greater levels of stimulation, and also for the positive and negative aspects of processor settings to be evaluated in the clinic and, if possible, assessed by parents, teachers and rehabilitation staff. An example of a programming schedule would be having a minimum of several sessions spread over 3 days for initial stimulation followed by programming sessions at 2 weeks, 1 month, 3 months, 6 months and a year post stimulation with 6-monthly sessions during the second and third years after stimulation. The process of adjustment to new stimulation and changes in programming can be facilitated by alternating rehabilitation sessions with tuning sessions. The cochlear implant team's rehabilitation staff can provide valuable feedback from their own observations and that of local professionals as to the benefit and progress made since the last tuning session, and this can supplement any more formal measures of the benefit obtained from the implant system in the clinic.

Assessing the benefit and efficacy of programming with a cochlear implant

Detailed assessment of the benefit of the cochlear implant system forms an integral part of the rehabilitation process. The ability of the child to use the implant to detect on/off, long/short, high and low frequency, and different speech sounds such as Ling's Five Sounds (Ling, 1975) need to be quantified. Ling's Five Sounds test can also be used as a quick daily test to check that the child is receiving a signal through the implant. Evans (1992) has described the test for checking the functioning of FM radio aid systems. With older children and those who have used their implant for longer periods of time, specific tests of speech discrimination and speech perception may be used as discussed by Beiter, Staller and Dowell (1991), Tyler (1993) and in Chapter 11. It is useful to include some assessment with the child using their implant as part of the programming of their device for the following reasons.

- To check that the child responds to sound using the implant.
- To assess any changes following adjustments to the programming of the processor.
- As a further check of loudness discomfort.
- To demonstrate to parents the auditory stimuli the child responds to when using the implant.

All of the above issues are important to obtain the best possible auditory input for the child and to reassure parents that their child is responding to sound. Children will often take the new sound sensation in their stride after an initial period of adjustment, and will not continually describe what they hear or even show demonstrable reaction to sound. In general, younger children are less likely to show active responses to sound. Adult implantees can describe what they hear and indicate whether or not the sound is pleasant. Adults are also aware that objects, such as the telephone or door bell, make sound whereas children have to learn to associate objects with environmental sounds. Adult implantees and older children with more recently acquired hearing losses will have sufficient language to describe the quality and quantity of the signal that they receive through their implants, and may be able to participate sufficiently in speech discrimination testing for the audiologist to be able to determine any improvements following the changes in processor settings. With young children with some limited

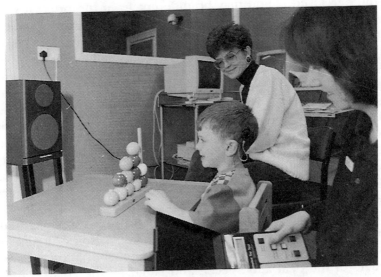

Figure 7.5 Photograph of a child undergoing aided sound field warble-tone testing using his cochlear implant

linguistic ability before implantation, the ideal would be to carry out a simple speech discrimination test which is a closed set test using seven paired toy items with similar vowel sounds but different consonants (McCormick, 1977), which is available in an automated form and can be calibrated (Ousey et al., 1989). In the author's own programme six children implanted at age 5 years or under required between 8 months and 2 years of time using their implant before they could obtain a score in the Automated IHR/McCormick speech toy discrimination test (Sheppard, Cope and Twomey, 1993). The fact that these children can carry out simple speech discrimination without lipreading is very rewarding and an excellent demonstration of the benefit of implantation. Before implanted children are able to carry out tests of this nature, different methods of measurement of detection of sound stimuli must be employed. Ling's Five Sounds can be used in a simple detection test with live voice. Sound detection can also be checked using warble-tone sound field measurements (Figure 7.5). Here the child is again conditioned to carry out a task, such as putting a man in a boat, when they hear a sound. This technique has the advantage that it is already very familiar to the child and information will be gained about broadly which frequencies and level of sound the child can detect – giving an early indication about which frequencies the child can detect with the implant. Caution must, however, be applied when using this type of measurement with a feature extraction processor such as the Nucleus device which is designed to process speech signals primarily. With this device, non-speech signals may be processed so that the perceived sound may be different from the original warble tone (Mecklenburg et al., 1990). Additionally the sensitivity setting of processors will affect the response level and should therefore be set at the optimum level which the child would normally use. Warble-tone measurements have nevertheless been successfully used to determine whether particular processor settings result in some frequencies being grossly more sensitive than others and whether specific frequency bands cause discomfort. This type of information is helpful in identifying which areas of the map or processor settings need further investigation; it is obtained when the child is unable to describe the quality of the sound signal through the implant or is unable to carry out the more sophisticated task of balancing or pitch ranking. It is still recommended, however, that these tasks are performed at a later stage.

Measurements carried out in the clinic can be supplemented by reports of implantees' performance in the field. Liaison with and information fed back from the implant team's rehabilitation personnel (teachers of the deaf and speech and language therapists), and the child's own teachers and parents, is valuable in assessing changes in processor settings. Changes in behaviour and changes in response to environmental and speech sounds may give indications to the audiologist about the efficacy of processor settings.

Guidance on the use of the implant equipment

Some time should be included in the programming sessions for each implanted child to discuss how the implant functions and the relationship between all the measurements carried out in the clinic and the functioning of the device. As both the programming and the device itself may appear complex, this education process needs to be ongoing for parents and visiting professionals. The benefits of giving parents a better understanding of the device, its programming and functioning include better use of the device by the child, encouragement for parents in continuing to have an active role in rehabilitation and more realistic expectations of their child's performance with an implant. Written information and diagrams could be useful to supplement information given verbally in the clinic.

On a more practical level, it is important that parents and local carers and professionals have a clear understanding of any control or function lights on the processor and how they should be set. It is obviously insufficient for the child to just wear the processor and headset; they must use them actively. For most of the time young children are in the care of their parents or teachers. It is therefore necessary for all adults involved with the child to know how to connect up the external components of the implant system correctly, so that they can change connecting cables if a fault is suspected. They also need to know how to clean and adjust the battery contacts safely when necessary. The Nucleus speech processor has 'M' and 'C' test lights. The 'M' light indicates battery charge, and also flashes when the processor is transmitting a signal in response to sound. The 'C' light indicates that the transmitter coil is emitting a signal if the coil is held against the centre of the processor. Parents and teachers should be encouraged to make use of the 'M' and 'C' lights to check the functioning of external equipment.

The switches or controls on most speech processors are similar. All have a power on/off switch which may incorporate options for testing the processor. There may also be an auxiliary input socket for use during programming or with auxiliary equipment. Some processors, but not all, have a volume control which will make sound louder for the implantee as the volume control is turned up in a similar way to a volume control on a conventional hearing aid or radio. For those with no user volume control the maximum loudness level is set internally using measurements carried out in programming sessions. All processors have sensitivity controls, the setting of which determines the quietest levels of sound that will be transmitted. Thus on a low sensitivity setting only louder sounds will be received by the internal stimulator and electrode array, whereas on a high sensitivity setting even very quiet sounds will be transmitted to the internal electrode array. If the sensitivity is set too low not all of the sounds of speech may be transmitted. If the sensitivity is set too high quieter sounds in the background may be emphasised and affect the users' ability to discriminate speech. It is usually better to have the processor set or programmed so that the volume control (if there is one), and the sensitivity switch, are not set to the extremes of the dial. Manufacturer's guidance on fitting and setting up processors should give some indication of optimum volume and sensitivity settings.

Adults and older children using implants may, with experience, want to adjust the sensitivity setting of their processor slightly according to their listening conditions; for example, they may wish to turn the sensitivity down when near traffic noise but they may wish to increase the sensitivity when listening to a quiet speaker in quiet surroundings.

Problem identification and solution

Just as young children are unable to describe what they can hear with their implant system, they may be unable to indicate when there is a fault with equipment, particularly if the fault affects sound quality rather than the signal being too loud or absent. A variety of signs could be an indication of change in the auditory stimulation that the child is receiving through the implant.

- Any signs of discomfort such as: removal of the transmitter coil or headset; crying; withdrawal; and touching the transmitter coil or side of the head.
- Visible damage to the processor, microphone, coil or leads.
- Any processor warning light not illuminating appropriately (microphone, M, and coil, C, lights on the Nucleus processor).
- Change in the child's general behaviour, e.g. naughtiness or avoiding communication.
- Unwillingness of the child to use or wear the processor or headset.
- Frequent damage to the processor or headset.
- Change in the child's ability to perceive or produce speech.
- Change in the child's responsiveness to environmental sounds.

Any of these factors could indicate the presence of a fault, although other influences in the child's life such as a change of family or school circumstances could also result in some of the listed behaviours. If there is any doubt about the functioning of the implant system then checks on equipment should be instigated without delay. The child's progress with the implant system and the development of auditory means of communication is dependent not only on the child being implanted and fitted with the external components of the device but also on the consistent daily use of the implant system. If a fault is suspected a logical approach to problem identification is helpful as shown in Figure 7.6.

Initially, leads, connections, batteries and battery contacts can be checked to see if the fault can be rectified simply by changing leads and/or the battery or by adjusting and cleaning battery contacts. This can be done outside the clinic by parents or teachers, providing they have been adequately informed as described earlier. If simple actions cannot resolve the problem, other components such as the transmitter coil, microphone and appropriately programmed speech processor should be replaced. It may be necessary to replace all external components if the location of the fault cannot be identified quickly. If replacement of the external equipment does not resolve any suspected fault, the child should visit the clinic to check the programming of the processor. If a child shows signs of discomfort when using their implant system, a clinic visit should be arranged without delay and the child should not use their processor until any problem has been resolved. During such a programming session the source of lack of stimulation or over stimulation needs to be identified.

Sound field warble-tone measurements can be used with the child using the processor to identify frequency regions where there is poor or no response or where there is discomfort. Measurements of threshold and most comfortable loudness levels can help to identify any electrodes that have developed faults or any areas of the child's MAP which

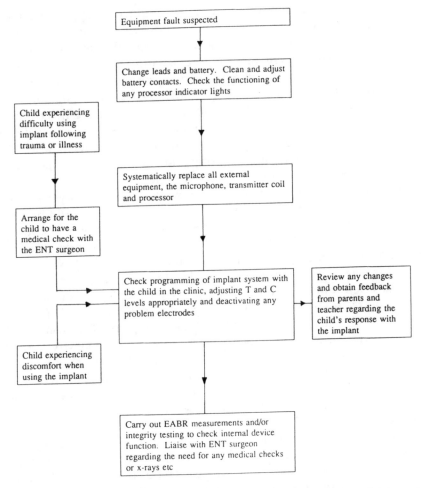

Figure 7.6 Flow diagram of a suggested method of identifying and resolving equipment and programming problems occurring in cochlear implant systems used by young children

may have altered since the previous session. The processor settings can be adjusted according to the changes in threshold and maximum comfortable loudness levels. Electrodes giving no response, aberrant measurements or discomfort should be deactivated. The child should be observed for signs of confusion or dislike during testing because this could indicate an electrode giving a poor or non-auditory response. Specific problems can be successfully identified and resolved by programming. It may not, however, be possible to identify any faults in a programming session if the child is too distressed to cooperate or if the stimulation is different and thus confusing to the child, resulting in variable threshold or maximum comfortable levels. Electrical auditory brain-stem response measurements can be used to investigate whether there is an auditory response to stimulation via the implant or the response through individual electrodes is suspected of malfunctioning. This type of measurement may require sedation and would be time-consuming to apply to all the electrodes of, for example, the Nucleus multichannel device, although it may nevertheless be invaluable in a situation where a clear picture cannot be obtained using behavioural techniques. If there has been any trauma or illness, it is advisable to involve medical and surgical members of the implant team who will examine the child; a radiograph (X-ray film) to check on the positioning of the electrode array may be recommended.

In the very rare situations where no comfortable auditory response can be restored the possibility of internal device failure should be considered. Some of the more recently designed implant systems have the facility to check the functioning of each internal electrode (Peeters, Offeciers and Marquet, 1990; Schindler and Kessler, 1992). With other devices it may be possible to carry out a test using scalp-recording electrodes to determine whether the internal receiver/stimulator is functioning and sending signals to the implanted electrodes. It is possible to do such an 'integrity test' with the Nucleus implant. With young children it would be advantageous to be able to do routine electrode function checks using electrodes and an oscilloscope to avoid unpleasant stimulation of a faulty electrode or time spent on trying to determine whether an electrode is giving some sound sensation or not (see Chapter 6). Internal device failures and reinsertions have been discussed in Chapter 5.

In the author's own clinic electrode failures with the Nucleus device are rare – only 13 electrodes in a series of 32 children, i.e. 2% of those implanted into the cochlea. For three electrodes in one child there was discomfort necessitating an emergency visit to the clinic. The remaining 10 electrodes in 6 children were discovered during routine programming sessions emphasising the need for follow-up checks on device functioning (Sheppard, Cope and Twomey, 1993).

Problems with discomfort or non-auditory sensations may also occur with partial insertion of the electrode array. This arises as a result of stimulation of non-auditory tissues outside the cochlea, because either the electrode stimulated is outside the cochlea or current is spreading to electrodes outside the cochlea. This type of problem may not be evident at initial tuning because of the limited number of electrodes used and the conservative dynamic ranges set. As the dynamic range increases, any problems with current spreading outside the cochlea will necessitate further adjustment to the map and reports from the surgeon regarding the depth of insertion of the electrode array can give helpful guidance. Any alterations to programming or deactivation of electrodes should be monitored and reviewed to ensure that the situation has stabilised and that no further reprogramming is required. Contact with parents and teachers in the interim period can give valuable information about the child's progress since programming changes have been made.

Use of auxiliary listening devices

The use of FM aids and connections to telephone, TV and radio all provide additional help for hearing-impaired children who use conventional hearing aids. The use of the auxiliary equipment provides the same pitfalls for implantees as for hearing aid users. The Nucleus system has an additional component known as the audio input selector which can be used to allow the implantee to listen using induction loop systems, including telephones fitted with an induction loop. Direct input systems with equipment such as TV, radio or music systems must be approached with caution with implantees and are not recommended where a direct connection is made between the implant and mains electricity. The advice of the implant manufacturers should be obtained with reference to the specific equipment that the implantee wishes to use.

The use of FM aids with children, particularly those whose educational setting is wholly or partially in mainstream school with poor acoustical conditions in the classroom, is an important issue. Wood, Cope and McCormick (1990), Lewis et al. (1991) and Ross (1992) have discussed in detail the setting up and use of FM aids with conventional hearing aids. The use of FM aids with the Nucleus implant has not been fully resolved because of the difficulty in achieving a direct input between the radio receiver and the speech processor, which gives a good signal without interference. This is thought to be the result of interference between the FM carrier frequency and the external equipment of the implant system, which uses a radio link to transmit the power and signal to the implanted receiver stimulator. This problem would not occur in systems with a percutaneous plug such as the Ineraid implant but, for reasons already discussed in Chapter 2, these are rarely used with children. Some implant systems have not been used extensively enough with children needing FM systems to know whether or not similar interference exists.

When using FM aids with conventional hearing aids, it is recommended that the hearing aid/FM aid system is set up individually for each child (Wood, Cope and McCormick, 1990). The same is true for FM aids and speech processors because the volume or balancing control of the FM system must be set so as to give a clear signal through the speech processor with the minimum interference or electrical noise. This must be done with the implantee and obviously cannot be carried out in a hearing aid test box. It may be feasible to set up an FM system with an adult and then test it with a child using a familiar auditory-only task under the conditions of use. By looking at the processor lights, it is possible to determine whether either a signal is being transmitted or there is a continuous noise if the M light remains on when there is no sound. Different designs of attenuation cable have been tried to couple the Nucleus processor to FM aids with some success (Heller and Shallop, 1993). With young children, however, or children unable to describe changes in the signal through their implant system, it is possible that an incorrectly set and connected FM aid could worsen the signal quality through the processor rather than improve the signal-to-noise ratio.

Radio aid use may result in the processor microphone being inactive and therefore the child will hear only the teacher and not any classmates. If the environmental microphone of the radio aid is used simultaneously with the transmitter input, background noise may be picked up by the environmental microphone while the teacher is speaking. The most recent models of radio aids incorporate a mute facility that mutes the environmental microphone automatically when a signal is detected by the radio transmitter which helps to overcome this problem.

Future developments in implant systems will, it is hoped, consider their use with FM systems more closely to help exclude any interfacing problems. In addition FM aids of the future may well be designed with both cochlear implantees and hearing aid users in mind because the numbers of children implanted is likely to grow rapidly. In the meantime it would be advisable to seek manufacturer's advice regarding suitable connection cables for FM systems and processors, and then to proceed with caution and close individual monitoring of each child in the classroom situation, so that any reduction in the quality of the signal can be identified.

Concluding remarks

Following the implantation of young children, rehabilitation and long-term maintenance of benefit is an integral process. There are two major components to the rehabilitation of implanted children: (1) the setting up or tuning of the device to suit each individual child and (2) encouragment of the child to use the new sound sensation. The better programmed the device, the more beneficial and time-effective the rehabilitation process will be. Early information about the child's use of sound stimulation will, however, also help the audiologist with fine tuning of the processor settings. This interactive process is necessary over an extended period of time, and even after the device has been optimally programmed contact with the audiology clinic will be required to rectify any problems. Long-term commitment is required to keep children consistently and efficiently using their implant systems throughout their lives.

Future developments in implant systems and the expansion of knowledge about implanted children will assist the process of programming implant systems for children. Implant systems may be developed with children in mind as users and may have options for easier early programming and facilitate the routine use of FM radio aids with cochlear implant systems. With greater knowledge it may be possible to predict advantageous changes in programming and identify potential difficulties earlier.

Acknowledgement

The study of intraoperative recordings of the EABR and ESRT in Nottingham has been supported financially by the Hearing Research Trust.

References

American Speech–Language–Hearing Association (1992). Electrical stimulation for cochlear implant selection and rehabilitation. *American Speech Language and Hearing Association*, **34** (Suppl. 7), 13–16.

Balkany, T., Gantz, B. and Nadol, J.B. (1988). Multichannel cochlear implants in partially ossified cochleas. *Annals of Otology, Rhinology and Laryngology*, **97**, 3–7.

Battmer, R.D., Laszig, R. and Lehnhardt, E. (1990). Electrically elicited stapedius reflex in cochlear implant patients. *Ear and Hearing*, **11** (5), 370–374.

Beiter, A.L., Staller, S.J. and Dowell, R.C. (1991). Education and device programming in children. *Ear and Hearing*, **12** (4) (Suppl), 25s–35s.

Boothroyd, A., Hanin, L., Yeung, E. and Chen, QY. (1992). Video-game for speech perception testing and training of young hearing impaired children. Proceedings of the John Hopkins National Search for Computer Applications to assist persons with disabilities, pp. 25–28. February 1–5, Laurel, Maryland, IEEE Computer Society Press, Los Almitos, California.

Burian, K., Hochmair-Desoyer, I.J. and Eisenwort, B. (1986). The Vienna cochlear implant programme. *Otolaryngology Clinics of North America*, **19**, 313–328.

Evans, C.H. (1992). Troubleshooting FM systems. In M. Ross (ed.), *FM Auditory Training Systems. Characteristics Selection and Use*, pp. 125–155. Simonium, MA: York Press.

George, C., Sheridan, C., Cafarelli Dees, D., Haacke, N.P., Worsfold, S. and Downie, A. (1993). Effect of duration of deafness (<2 years vs >20 years) on performance and preferred stimulation with Nucleus 22-channel cochlear implant. Paper presented at the 3rd International Cochlear Implant Conference, April 4–7 1993, Innsbruck, Austria.

Heller, J.W. and Shallop, J.K. (1993). Use of FM assistive listening systems with cochlear implants. Paper presented at the 3rd International Cochlear Implant Conference, April 4–7 1993, Innsbruck, Austria.

Hochmair-Desoyer, I.J. (1986). Fitting of an analogue cochlear prothesis–introduction of a new method and preliminary findings. *British Journal of Audiology*, **20**, 45–53.

Hortman, G., Pulec, J.L., Causse, J.B., Causse, J.R., Briend, C., Fontaine, J.P., Tetu, F. and Azema, B. (1989). Experience with the extracochlear multichannel Implex system. In B. Fraysse (ed.), *Cochlear Implant Acquisitions and Controversies*, pp. 307–317. Basel: Cochlear. (Manuscript of International Symposium Toulouse, June 9–10 1989).

Kerber, M., Herka, H. and Klasek, O. (1993). Straightforward approach to fitting for the MED-EL speech processor with children. Paper presented at the Third International Cochlear Implant Conference, Innsbruck, Austria, April.

Lewis, D.E., Feigin, J.A., Karasek, A.E. and Stelmachowicz, P. G. (1991). Evaluation and assessment of FM systems. *Ear and Hearing* 12, 268–280.

Ling, D. (1975). Evaluation, other aspects of evaluation. *Speech and the Hearing Impaired Child: Theory and Practices*, pp. 157–159.

MacPherson, B.J., Elfenbein, J.L., Schum, R.L. and Bentler, R.A. (1991). Thresholds of discomfort in young children. *Ear and Hearing*, 12, 184–190.

McCormick B. (1977). The Toy Discrimination Test: An aid for screening the hearing of children above a mental age of 2 years. *Public Health*, 91, 67–73.

McCormick, B. (ed.) (1988). Behavioural hearing tests, 6 months to 5 years. In *Paediatric Audiology: 0–5 Years*, pp. 97–116. London: Whurr.

Mason, S.M., Sheppard, S., Garnham, C.W., Lutman, M.E., O'Donoghue, G.M. and Gibbin, K.P. (1994). Application of intra-operative recordings of electrically evoked auditory brainstem responses in a paediatric cochlear implant programme. *Proceedings of the International Symposium on Cochlear Implants – New Perspectives*, in press. Toulouse, France, June 2–3 1992.

Mecklenburg, D.J., Blamey, P.J., Busby, P.A., Dowell, R.C., Roberts, S. and Rickards, F.W. (1990). Auditory (re)habilitation for implanted deaf children and teenagers. In G.M. Clark, Y.C. Tong and J.F. Patrick (eds), *Cochlear Protheses*, pp. 207–221. London: Churchill Livingstone.

Osberger, M.J., Todd, S.L., Robbins, A.M., Berry, S.W. and Miyamoto, R.T. (1991). Effect of age at onset of deafness on children's speech perception abilities with a cochlear implant. *Annals of Otology, Rhinology and Laryngology*, 100, 883–888.

Ousey, J., Sheppard, S., Twomey, T., and Palmer, A.R. (1989). The IHR/McCormick Toy Discrimination Test – description and initial evaluation. *British Journal of Audiology*, 23, 245–251.

Patrick, J.F. and Clark, G.M. (1991). The Nucleus 22-channel cochlear implant system. *Ear and Hearing*, 12, (4), 35–95.

Parkin, J. and Stewart, B.E. (1988). Multichannel cochlear implantation: Utah-design. *The Laryngoscope*, 98, 262–265.

Patrick. J.F., Seligman, P.M., Money, D.K. and Kuzma, J.A. (1990). Engineering. In G.M. Clark, Y.C. Tong and J.F. Patrick (eds), *Cochlear Protheses*, pp. 99–124. London: Churchill Livingstone.

Peeters, S., Offeciers, F.E. and Marquet, J.F.E. (1990). The Laura Cochlear Prothesis: technical aspects. In T. Sacriotan, J.J. Alvares-Vocent, J. Bartual, F. Antole-Condela et al. (eds), *Otorhinolaryngology, Head and Neck Surgery*. 1989, Amsterdam: Kugler and Ghedini.

Pfingst, B.E., Spelman, F.A., and Sutton, D. (1980). Operating ranges for cochlear implants. *Annals of Otology and Rhinology, Laryngology*, 89 (Suppl. 66), 1–4.

Roberts, S. (1991). Speech processor fitting for cochlear implants. In H. Cooper (ed.), *Cochlear Implants: A Practical Guide*, pp. 201–218. London: Whurr.

Ross, M. (1992). *FM Auditory Training Systems. Characteristics, Selection and Use*. Timonium, MA: York Press.

Schindler, R.A. and Kessler, D.K. (1992). Preliminary results with the Clarion cochlear implant. *The Laryngoscope*, **102**, 1006–1013.

Shallop, J.K., Beiter, A.L., Goin, D.W. and Mischke, R.E. (1990). Electrically evoked auditory brainstem responses (EABR) and middle latency responses (EMLR) obtained from patients with the Nucleus multichannel cochlear implant. *Ear and Hearing*, **11** (1), 5–15.

Shallop, J.K., Goin, D.W., Van Dyke, L. and Mischke, R.E. (1991). Prediction of behavioural threshold and comfort values for Nucleus 22 channel implant patients from electrical auditory brainstem response test results. *Annals of Otology, Rhinology and Laryngology*, **100**, 896–898.

Sheppard, S., Cope, Y and Twomey, T. (1993). Programming the Nucleus 22 channel cochlear implant for young children: Issues and problems. Proceedings of the 3rd International Cochlear Implant Conference, April 4–7 1993, Innsbruck, Austria, in press.

Staller, S.J., Beiter, A.L. and Brimacombe, J.A. (1991). Children and multichannel cochlear implants. In H. Cooper (ed.), *Cochlear Implants: A Practical Guide*, pp. 283–321. London: Whurr.

Staller, S., Beiter, A.L., Brimacombe, J.A., Mecklenburg, D.J. and Arnolt, P. (1991). Paediatric performance with the Nucleus 22 channel cochlear implant system. *American Journal of Otology*, **12** (Suppl.), 126–136.

Stephan, K., Welzl-Muller, K. and Stiglbrumer, H. (1991). Acoustic reflex in patients with cochlear implants (analog stimulation). *American Journal of Otology*, **12** (Suppl.), 48–51.

Tye-Murray, N. (1993). Aural rehabilitation and patient management. In R.S. Tyler (ed.), *Cochlear Implants: Audiological Foundations*, pp. 87–144. London: Whurr.

Tyler, R.S. (1993). Speech perception by Children. In R.S. Tyler (ed.), *Cochlear Implants: Audiological Foundations*, pp. 191–256. London: Whurr.

von Wallenberg, E.L. and Battmer, R.D. (1991). Comparative speech recognition results in eight subjects using two different coding strategies with the Nucleus 22 channel cochlear implant. *British Journal of Audiology*, **25**, 371–380.

Wood, S.A. (1988). Pure tone audiometry. In B. McCormick (ed.), *Paediatric Audiology 0–5 Years*, pp. 137–166. London: Whurr.

Wood, S., Cope, Y. and McCormick, B. (1990). A guide to fitting type 2 Radio Hearing Systems in direct input mode. *Journal of the British Association of Teachers of the Deaf*, **(14)** (5), 133–141.

Chapter 8
Rehabilitation: a practical approach

SUE ARCHBOLD and MARGARET TAIT

This chapter describes briefly some rehabilitation approaches for children with cochlear implants, and goes on to describe practical activities which have been found useful in facilitating the use of the implant system.

Is rehabilitation necessary for children with cochlear implants?

The aim in rehabilitating young children with cochlear implants is to enable them to learn to listen to the new sensations of sounds, to attach meaning to them and to use their hearing in the development of spoken language. In the case of a hearing child, the usual route by which communication skills, and hence spoken language, are acquired is audition. A child who is audiologically appropriate for implantation will not have been receiving any significant benefit from hearing aids, and will have relied for communication upon vision (whether by lipreading or signing). Implantation can provide useful hearing for many of these children (Boothroyd, 1991; McCormick, 1991), and the child will need to learn to interpret and integrate the sound signals received in order to communicate effectively. Is it enough then to provide useful hearing and let the usual pattern of development take place? For a child who has been without significant audition for some time, one needs to 'Make the normal happen' (Tait, 1987), i.e. provide the situations which are known to facilitate the development of spoken language in both hearing and deaf children. To maximise the benefits from the implant system, the children need the following:

- Wearing of the device all waking hours, in good working order.
- Appropriate tuning of the device for the child.

- Good listening conditions, bearing in mind the difficulties of learning to listen in conflicting background noise.
- Opportunities for non-linguistic listening experiences.
- Opportunities to develop appropriate communication skills in adult–child, child–child and adult–children interactions.
- Experience of success in developing listening and communication skills in age-appropriate interactions.
- Cooperation of all involved with the child: parents, siblings, peers, teachers, speech and language therapists, and any other carers.

These requirements are not so different from those appropriate for young children who wear conventional acoustic hearing aids. The rehabilitation activities described in this chapter are similar to those used with hearing-aided children and are based on ideas developed with such children over many years, which experienced teachers of the deaf will recognise. However, while relying on experiences with hearing-aided children, some differences are worth noting in working with children with cochlear implants:

- The complexity of tuning the device.
- The complexity of monitoring device functioning.
- The sudden onset of audition after a long period with no useful auditory input.
- The necessity to help the child use audition as effectively and quickly as possible.
- The expectation of greater access to mid and high-frequency information than is usual with conventional hearing aids.

Whether rehabilitation is necessary for children following implantation has been a subject for debate with few hard data to determine whether rehabilitation programmes have been effective, or if one method is more effective than another in adults or children (Cooper, 1991). Children receiving implants should already have been the subject of specialised education before implantation and, after implantation, although educational placement and communication styles (whether oral or total communication) may initially remain the same (Tye-Murray, 1993), the consensus of opinion is that a strong auditory/oral component is essential to optimise the use of the implant (Cooper, 1991; Somers, 1991; Tye-Murray, 1993). Boothroyd (1989) gives two prerequisites for the use of audition in the development of spoken language: the provision of suitable amplification and the provision of suitable training. An emphasis on audition may well have been inappropriate before implantation, but once useful hearing has been provided by an implant, then appropriate training must begin. Those children receiving implants will have experienced failure in the use of hearing (Somers, 1991), and the implant team must implement a rehabilitation programme which will enable the child to develop confidence in his or her new auditory skills as soon as possible. As Osberger (1990) states: 'there is no question that rehabilitation is an essential part of paediatric implant work.' There is also no question that, as described in Chapter 3, this rehabilitation must be in close liaison with the child's parents and local educators, who will bear the main responsibility for developing the child's use of the system. The rehabilitation must not, however, be at the expense of the other deaf children in the educator's care; it may well be that, following implantation, the child will not receive more time than before, but that the time spent with him or her will have a different focus: the development of the use of audition.

Approaches to rehabilitation

Having established that these children need rehabilitation following implantation, what form should it take? Although many of the issues surrounding work with deaf children are old, cochlear implantation opened a new chapter in the saga, with discussion about the most effective way to maximise the use of audition. Techniques used with children with cochlear implants include multisensory or unisensory training, synthetic or analytical training, unstructured or structured methods. These theoretical frameworks are described elsewhere (Eisenberg, 1985; Cooper, 1991; Somers, 1991; Tye-Murray, 1993); the aim here is not to add to the conflict, but briefly to consider what is known of children's learning, whether deaf or hearing, and how this knowledge can influence rehabilitation.

The quality of adult–child interaction and the importance of meaning within early language learning experience is vital (Bruner,1983); the adult must be responsive to the child's attempts at communication, to facilitate the development of language, rather than imposing the adult's interests on the child (Webster, 1992). Emphasis on the repetition of the adult's contribution, the correction of the child's own contribution and on adult questioning have been found to be counterproductive to the development of communication skills, and hence language, in both hearing and hearing-impaired children (Wood et al., 1986). This theme will be developed further as the acquisition of communication skills in children at the pre-verbal stage is discussed. Highly structured, adult-controlled methods of promoting the use of the device are contrary to what we know facilitates communication and linguistic development in both hearing and hearing-impaired children. The emphasis on an analytical (or bottom-up) approach to rehabilitation relies on training children in specific goals within the clinic, assuming that a skill learned will be generalised into everyday life. The approach developed in Nottingham tends towards the synthetic (or top-down) approach in which children learn to use hearing in natural situations, discovering the rules of communication for themselves and becoming able to use their useful hearing in the development of language. The adult's role is not that of a mere observer, however, but that of a vital facilitator of the child's learning; the adult must structure the learning experiences for the child, bearing in mind an overview of the likely sequence of development of auditory skills and leading the child on to the next stage of development (Webster, 1992).

Tye-Murray (1993) considers four influences on the aural rehabilitation programme for an implantee: (1) the design of the implant being used, (2) the tuning of the device, (3) theories of listening development and (4) knowledge of patients' abilities with an implant. With these influences in mind, some practical activities have been developed which help with the following:

- Development of the child's attachment of meaning to sound.
- Development of the child's reliance on audition.
- Development of the child's listening skills.
- Development of the use of audition in the development of communication and spoken language skills.

In addition, these activities help to monitor the functioning and tuning of the implant system. Before a programme of suitable activities can be initiated, however, the implant system must be managed appropriately.

Managing the implant system

For rehabilitation to be effective, the child must be wearing the device adjusted comfortably at appropriate settings. This implies that the audiological scientist has been able to tune the system optimally, and that the child has accepted the device and the new sensations of sound. In practice this may be far from straightforward, particularly with young children. The tuning of the device, described fully in Chapter 7, may take several visits to the clinic over a period of some time. The child may not accept the new sensation happily, and it may be necessary to progress slowly in small steps until the optimum program for the processor is achieved. This will require the combined skills of the family and the local and implant professionals. Fryauf-Bertschy (1992) gives practical advice to parents about the preparation for the initial tuning session; it is useful if the child has seen others wearing the device, and has tried on the dummy processor and headset, to ensure that he or she can wear it comfortably before receiving the signal. Fryauf-Berstchy (1992) also gives practical ideas for wearing the processor, and for encouraging children who may reject it. Children may reject the implant system and its signal for many reasons; it may have been inappropriately tuned, but at an experienced centre this should be rare. It may be that the child is disturbed by the new sensation, or it may be that the child realises that the attitude to the implant system gives him or her a powerful manipulative weapon to use. Children may be more tired, or more distractible, than usual after the initial tuning; some have been known to have nightmares after the onset of audition.

It is important that parents and local educators know that, although many children accept the onset of audition happily, adverse reactions are possible. They should feel supported by, and have confidence in, the implant team in their efforts to encourage wearing of the device. From the beginning, children should wear the implant system for the whole day; it may be necessary at first to turn the system off or adjust the controls in noisy conditions, in the car or shop, for example, but this is less disruptive for a young child than taking the system off and putting it on again. The child should not, initially, be given use of the controls, but realise that the parent or teacher takes responsibility for adjusting the controls if necessary.

Constant use of the system is only effective if the device is functioning optimally. Handbooks for the Nucleus processor are produced by Cochlear AG, and at the authors' programme parents and teachers are given a simple trouble-shooting guide and spare leads to keep at home and at school. It is essential that, in addition to carrying out a daily check of the signal through the processor, parents and professionals quickly recognise any changes in the subtle signs which reveal auditory awareness on the part of the child. The rehabilitation ideas in this chapter, as well as being designed to promote listening skills in pleasurable ways, are suitable for providing situations in which an observant parent or professional can monitor device functioning. Intermittent faults with the system can be particularly difficult to pinpoint, and may only be noticed when a child appears confused in a listening activity within his or her capabilities. The listening activities which are described in this chapter follow a hierarchy of developing skills, and are described under the headings of the functional classification that the authors use for their children. These categorisations are first outlined.

Categorisation of implanted children

For reasons described in Chapter 11, the Nottingham programme uses a functional classification, rather than an aetiological one, and children are categorised by their linguistic functioning at the time of implantation so that developments can be assessed from this baseline.

The following functional classification (discussed more fully in Chapter 11) is used:

Pre-verbal	to describe those children with few, or none, of the early communication skills which are the precursors of spoken language
Transitional	to describe those children beginning to use sound in a meaningful way for communication
Functional spoken language	to describe those children who are beginning to use oral language as a primary means of everyday communication

A linguistic classification has been helpful in monitoring progress of the children through these stages, and in deciding which activities and tests are appropriate. The rest of this chapter is devoted to describing some of the practical activities found useful in promoting the use of audition after implantation. They are described under the headings: 'Working with pre-verbal children', 'Working with children at the transitional stage' and 'Working with children with functional language'.

At each stage activities will be outlined which develop listening to environmental sounds, to musical instruments and to spoken language; they are not mutually exclusive, and can be adapted for use in different educational settings. They emphasise the development of listening throughout the child's day, not only in the implant clinic, and should be used with care in interactive situations. First a description is given for those suitable for children at the pre-verbal stage.

Working with pre-verbal children

The aim with children at the pre-verbal level is to work with parents and teachers to facilitate the development of communication. Once they have been implanted and fitted with the speech processor and headset, they will be in a similar position to that of acoustic hearing aid users – that is, with the potential of using their hearing. However, before they begin to understand what is said to them, and to use speech themselves, there needs to be development of the pre-verbal skills of appropriate eye contact, turn-taking, auditory processing and meaningful vocalisation (see Chapter 10 on video analysis for fuller discussion). Below are some guidelines on helpful approaches with pre-verbal children, and also some practical suggestions. They are described with reference to developing eye contact, turn-taking and auditory processing; in addition, suggestions for the development of meaningful vocalisations and the use of singing at the pre-verbal stage are included. For simplification, the adult is referred to throughout as 'she' and the child as 'he'.

Developing eye contact and turn-taking at the pre-verbal stage

A deaf child in the very earliest stage of language development is likely to be unaware of the adult's attempts to communicate with him: to be 'disengaged' (Tait, 1987). Strategies which at a later stage might be of some use to attract his attention, or to indicate that a contribution from him is expected, will probably not be helpful with a child who is not engaged in the interaction.

For example, holding an object up to the mouth while speaking is likely to remove the natural clues to the meaning of what is said. It is not possible to 'make' the young pre-verbal child 'understand' in this way. He may follow the object with his eyes – particularly if he was already playing with it and the adult has taken it away from him to say something about it – but the adult's utterance will not have meaning for him. Similarly, one cannot 'make' him communicate, and efforts to do this are likely to be unproductive. An approach which expects the child to attend to and interpret what is in the adult's mind is asking something of the child that he is not capable of giving at this stage. The initial approach to a pre-verbal child needs to be on the lines of the mother with her hearing baby. The adult needs to follow the child's line of gaze and comment on what he is looking at, even though at first he will probably be unaware of her. In other words, the adult needs to interpret what is in the child's mind and not the other way about. This is not to say, however, that the child is allowed to choose what to do all the time.

The use of partner and parallel play

There are several ways of making the adult's presence interesting to a child at the pre-verbal stage. One answer is to become a partner – but the *less dominant* partner – in play, for example, to be the patient to the child's doctor, the hungry person at the table waiting for the child to serve the dinner, the visitor knocking to be let in, and so on. It is at times such as these that the presence of another adult can be invaluable. One adult can be the naughty patient refusing medicine, while the other arouses interest in her and helps the doctor to administer suitable treatment.

Another way is to play 'in parallel' with an unresponsive child. Parallel play is a stage which normally comes between solitary and cooperative play. Children engage in the same activity, side by side, each of them modifying what he is doing because of the actions of the other child, though not actually playing *with* the other child. This form of play has been observed to occur much more rarely with hearing-impaired children (Gross, 1987), and that may well be because they have less auditory feedback to let them know what the child playing alongside is doing and planning to do. They therefore simply play alongside until they reach the stage of being able to join in cooperative play. For the adult to be the parallel (but again subordinate) partner in play can be a good way of promoting interaction in an unstressful, uncontrolling manner. One simply engages in the same activity that has been chosen by the child – for example, playing with pastry – and does whatever the child does. Before long he becomes aware of this, and observes the adult's actions as well as his own, sometimes deliberately egging her on by unexpected behaviour (putting pastry on his nose, for example), thus giving lots of opportunities for one-to-one conversation and interaction dominated by the child.

The use of familiar formats

The establishment of some 'format' (see Chapter 10) which catches the child's interest (and, if possible, causes amusement) is in the authors' experience the most likely way of enabling appropriate eye contact and turn-taking to develop. An example follows from a one-to-one session with a profoundly deaf boy aged 3 years, who at this period had very little receptive or expressive language. The adult's (A) and child's (C) 'turns' are presented in sequence. Notes on gestures and focus of visual attention are given in round brackets for the adult and square brackets for the child:

A: That's it! You're driving your car, and then we stop (sitting back), don't we, stop (policeman's 'stop' gesture), like that. [C looks at A throughout, until A gestures, then glances at gesture, and back at A].

C: [Gestures 'stop', glancing at his gesturing hand, and back at A].

A: Stop, the policeman says (glances at her hand), Stop! (with gesture), doesn't he. [C looks at A, then follows her glance at her hand by looking at both hands, and back at her.]

C: (st)o(p) [said without voice, with gesture, and a look at their gestures].

A: Stop. Yes, and then he says – (her arm is moving in preliminary to gesture) – Go! (gesture). [C has looked at her gesture preliminary, but looks back at her as she says Go.]

C: (g)o! [gesturing].

A: Go, that's right, and we'll drive our cars again.

As this little routine is familiar to the child, it is very clear to him where his 'turn' comes. He is able *to take* his 'turn' first by gesture, then by gesture and a silent attempt at the appropriate word, and finally by a vocal attempt. This is very much the sort of process followed by the normally hearing infant in well-known format-like routines.

Here is another example with a different child of the same age and similar hearing loss, from a session during which he has not looked at the adult at all. The child's attention is caught fleetingly by a nearby drum. The adult gives it to him to bang, and momentarily hangs on to his hand while she feigns 'sleep'. She releases his hand, whereupon he immediately hits the drum, and she 'wakes up'. This sequence is repeated several times. Because he is doing (or, more accurately, being helped to do) something which is fun for him, and which has an amusing result, his gaze for those few moments rests either on the adult or on the drum, instead of moving fleetingly around the room (Wood et al.,1986).

The use of shared activities

Appropriate patterns of eye contact – looking at the speaker, or at the object of discourse – and of turn-taking are stages of the child's development. They cannot be imposed on him. What one *can* do is to provide situations where there will be some point in his looking at the person communicating with him and in taking his turn in the interaction. The shared activity (making a paper puppet) described below, and illustrated in Figure 8.1, is an example which shows how this might happen in practice.

Briefly, the puppet is made as follows: rolled-up newspaper, pushed through a cardboard tube middle 'body', forms arms and legs; a screwed-up newspaper ball forms the head, with tissue paper wrapped round the head and thrust into the cardboard middle to form a connecting neck and also to provide a surface for a face. There are many opportunities in the shared making of this puppet for mutual gaze and turn-taking to develop. Imagine that the adult and child are facing each other across a small table as they begin. Instead of rolling up the newspaper to form the second arm/leg, the adult just struggles to push it through the cardboard tube middle unrolled. The child is likely to be keen to let her know her mistake, and to show what should be done. If the adult *pauses* momentarily in her activity – seizing up the action and

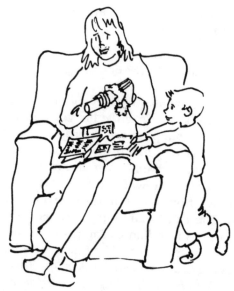

Figure 8.1 An example of a shared activity: puppet making

looking towards the child – he will probably take the opportunity to put her right, and will look at her to make sure she recognises her error and has received the instruction. Anyone with an important message to communicate wants to know that the message is being received! Appropriate response and facial expression on the adult's part will make the most of the incident.

This is only one fairly crude example. The most important thing in all encounters is for the adult to be aware of any glances that come her way, to recognise the reason, and act contingently (Wood et al.,1986). Any move a child makes toward the adult – and a glance in her direction is such a move – must be interpreted as communication and responded to as such. Similarly, one should treat any vocalisation as intentional communication and respond to it, just as the mother of the normally hearing baby does, leaving pauses in the utterances that are long enough and frequent enough for the child to have a chance to take part. It is especially important to respond to any vocalisation that the child makes during the adult's turn, and to relinquish one's own turn immediately. If a child takes a turn that has not been offered, it should be given to him. If many turns go by without his being able to take them, a brief return to a situation which he *can* recognise – a format – will help him get back into the conversation. This may take the form of a familiar 'joke', as in the next transcript in which the adult's (A) and the child's (C) turns are presented in sequence. Notes on the child's gestures are made in the square brackets.

A: I like this jumper. This is a lovely one.
C: [points at the stripes]
A: Yes, that's very nice. It's got yellow stripes.
   I would like that one, can I have it.
C: Mine!
A: You have this, and I'll have that!
C: [grins and shakes head]

Turn-taking is easier when the situation is predictable, which is why familiar formats and jokes play such an important part. Potentially fruitful activities are:

- playing with farm animals
- playing with road and cars
- cooking (real or pretend)
- model making
- looking at pop-up books
- cleaning shoes – or anything else
- washing anything
- setting the table
- any games/activities that involve an element of surprise, such as items hidden in a bag.

Developing auditory processing: helping children to use their hearing at the pre-verbal stage

It is important not to give children the impression that 'listening' is something that only happens at special times. There are advantages, however, in sound-making sessions whose main purpose is to make listening something that is exciting and fun. In the early days after initial tuning of the device, the easiest activity for a child is to perceive the onset of sound because *he* is producing the sound himself and can observe its effects on others. For example, he plays percussion instruments and the adult reacts – perhaps marching while he plays a drum, and falling over when he hits the cymbal, without looking at the child. The role of listener rather than producer of the sound need not be passive, for instance, the child hiding inside the playhouse and bursting forth when he has heard the sound. Similarly, it is great fun for him to listen for a sound and then send a skittle flying across the room (Figure 8.2).

These are very simple examples, and there are many more adventurous things that can be done using more sophisticated instruments, but the basic idea *is* simple: the child makes a sound and observes its effect on other people. He sees these other people react to the sound he is making even when they are not looking at him. Also, he begins to be

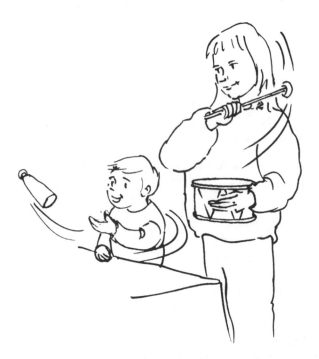

Figure 8.2 Developing a response to sound

aware of sound, and of the person making it, when *he* is not looking at the sound source.

Although the child's auditory attention may be caught initially by the use of musical and environmental sounds, what one particularly wants him to be aware of is the human voice. Again, a child who is not a ready vocaliser may begin by simply using his voice to 'operate' the adult. For example, the adult may curl up in a comfortable chair, while the child attempts to 'wake' her or get her moving by vocalising, illustrated in Figure 8.3. Then roles can be reversed so that the child is doing the listening.

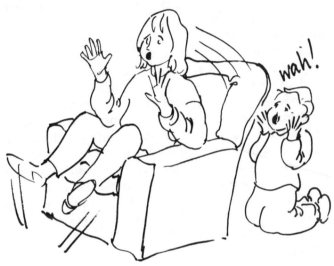

Figure 8.3 Learning to use voice to produce an effect

The role of singing with pre-verbal children

Singing is another activity that promotes listening, and also goes a long way towards solving many of the early problems with eye contact, turn-taking and vocalisation. The idea of singing with a child who is not yet talking may seem a surprising one, but in fact it is in many ways easier for a young deaf child than conversation. This is because some of the 'rules' and conventions of spoken exchanges are waived in this activity. Eye contact, for example, is more straightforward in a simple action song, because the child does not need to look anywhere else for information to understand what is going on. Similarly, vocalising comes more readily during singing because of there is no need for turn-taking. As eye contact and turn-taking are pre-verbal skills which one is trying to develop, an activity that encourages both in an enjoyable way is valuable. It has been found that young deaf children (wearing conventional hearing aids) at the pre-verbal stage maintain twice as much eye contact during the singing of simple action songs as they do during one-to-one conversational sessions with a known adult. With children at this stage there is seven times as much vocalisation in singing, compared with the talking situation. Additional benefits are that the children's voices are more varied in pitch and their utterances longer and more rhythmic (Tait, 1984). For all these reasons, singing is an activity to be recommended for all young children with implants, at any stage of their linguistic development, but particularly during the pre-verbal period.

The adult interacting with the child in singing needs to enjoy it and accept that being in tune is not important. What is important is to be near enough to be properly heard and seen, to sing at a reasonable volume and speed (not too slowly) and with rhythm. It is not necessary to try to get a very young child to watch the singer – he or she will probably watch if it is sufficiently interesting, and will be more likely to if the singer is enjoying it, because enjoyment is very contagious. On the other hand, a child who is not looking may possibly be listening, particularly if he or she is showing signs of being involved in what is going on – vocalising, for example, or doing the song actions. Similarly, it is better not to insist that the child joins in; singing should be an enjoyable experience. In additional, children are most vocal under conditions of least control (Wood et al., 1986) and they will be more likely to join in positively, take the lead and suggest songs themselves if they are not pressured (Tait, 1984). Tapes of appropriate songs and suggestions for their use are available from the Nottingham programme.

To summarise: during the pre-verbal stage development of the following is taking place:

- appropriate eye-contact
- conversational turn-taking
- meaningful vocalisation
- auditory processing.

Once these skills are becoming established, the children will start to understand speech and how to use vocalisations and speech sounds in communication in a meaningful way; they are considered to have moved on to the transitional stage, where other activities may become more appropriate.

Working with children at the transitional stage

At the pre-verbal stage the emphasis was on the development of early communication skills; at the transitional stage, when the child has some communication abilities and is beginning to respond, more structured activities to promote listening are possible. By this stage, there is awareness of voice and sounds in meaningful situations and some idea of the use of language, and of the underlying rules of communication.

Response to a variety of musical sounds, environmental sounds and speech sounds will be promoted; once observed, the ability to discriminate one sound from another will be encouraged. Discrimination will develop between sounds that are:

- loud or quiet
- single or repeated
- long or short
- high or low.

Discrimination will also develop between:

- different environmental sounds
- different musical instruments
- different speech sounds.

In planning appropriate activities for a child within these areas, there may be great disparity between the child's linguistic age and chronological age. For a child deaf from birth or deafened at an early age, and implanted some years later, it may be taxing to find age-appropriate and interest-appropriate tasks. This is a common problem when working with deaf children, but with children who have not had any useful hearing for a number of years the problem may be even greater. The sudden acquisition of useful hearing after a number of years without audition will necessitate a number of adjustments for both the child and his carers. Those interacting with the child on a daily basis must change their expectations, while not subjecting the child to any pressure to 'perform'. This demands quite subtle changes of handling on the part of parents and educators if the best possible use is to be made of the implant system.

Listening to environmental sounds at the transitional stage

For some, environmental sound discrimination is not an important part of the rehabilitation programme, but often the first observed responses are to environmental sounds, and it may be a major aim of implantation for safety reasons for parents (Eisenberg, 1985). At the transitional and functional language stage the children enjoy 'listening' walks, indoors and out, responding to environmental sounds and drawing pictures of those that they can hear. The sounds within home or clinic can be used so that the child becomes aware of the diversity of sounds around and begins the early stages of discrimination. When a child has shown his first response to sound for many years, it is very easy to be too keen to test his listening skills, and he will soon not wish to cooperate. Opportunities for drawing attention to sounds in the environment must be made and taken casually without putting the child under any pressure. Saying 'There's the doorbell – let's go and see who's there', rather than questioning the child as to what made the sound, helps him to attach meaning to the sound in a relaxed way. Picture books which illustrate sounds in the environment and stories which refer to sound are all appropriate for this stage, helping the child to relate meaning to the new sensations being received. Picture cards showing sounds in the child's environment are readily available, and home-made picture books can be coloured and completed as responses to sounds are observed. This may be helpful in demonstrating new listening skills to parents at a time when apparent progress may be slow.

Listening to musical instruments at the transitional stage

Although play with musical instruments will have formed part of the rehabilitation work with children at the pre-verbal stage, at the transitional and functional language stages it can be taken further. The term 'musical instruments' covers a wide range of sound makers. Fun may be had with toys which make a variety of sounds, noisy toy animals and a whole range of sound-making equipment. The children develop the games played at the pre-verbal stage, for example, moving or responding to different musical instruments in a variety of ways, and playing musical statues or hide-and-seek in response to sound.

Once responses in play have been observed to a variety of musical instruments, then discrimination can begin. Naturally discrimination games are started with musical instruments that are very dissimilar in sound, progressing to those that are more closely related. Children enjoy pretending to sleep and identifying the instrument which woke them up; different instruments can be played out of sight and the child can go to find them. Different ways in which instruments may be played can be introduced, for instance, the sound can be made louder as the child gets nearer and quieter as the child goes further away. Children enjoy imitation games as rhythm and intensity are altered, and pairs of instruments enable the adult and child to play alongside as imitative skills develop. Picture cards which illustrate different instruments and the differing ways in which they can be played should be devised, for example, the three cards illustrated in Figure 8.4 show a loud, a quiet and a silent drum.

Children at this stage become more able to join in conventional songs and rhymes at school, and teachers of the deaf often comment that a child is more able to participate in these activities following implantation, enjoying the repetitive songs which form part of the daily school routine. As with hearing-aided children, children with cochlear implants will often join in the repeated chorus of a well-known song, and many action rhymes enable children to respond with appropriate actions within a group (Figure 8.5), demonstrating developing listening skills, before they are able to join in the singing at all.

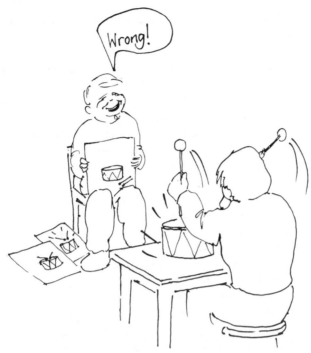

Figure 8.4 Picture cards can illustrate the different ways in which instruments are played, for example, a loud drum, a quiet drum and a silent drum

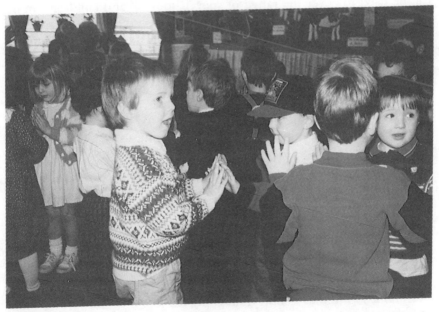

Figure 8.5 Children with cochlear implants benefit very much from joining in action songs with their peers

Listening to speech sounds: developing responses in play at the transitional stage

Initially a variety of action toys will be useful in producing a reaction to speech sounds and an observable response from the child. Wind up toys which have to be told to 'go' and 'stop' are useful. The adult makes a sound to accompany their progress, for example the monkey goes 'oo oo', the mouse goes 'ee ee'. These action toys interest a wide age range of children and provide opportunity for repetitive sound making, encouraging recognition and imitation of speech sounds without stress.

Animals, vehicles, puppets and action toys give opportunities for hearing and making speech sounds in game formats. For example, jumping toy frogs into the pond on vocal command, or play with farm animals, provide situations in which the child can hear and attempt to produce these sounds many times over in highly motivated situations. The animals can hide, pop out, go to market in turn in the lorry (accompanied by 'brmm brmm') and then settle down to sleep ('shh'). There are many books about animals that are appropriate for this stage and those that contain pictures for the child to open are most useful to encourage shared conversation and develop responses to speech sounds; these responses may initially be subtle, and may only be observable on video.

Animal sounds have the advantage that with a bit of ingenuity they can be used to cover the range of speech sounds, and children can be conditioned to associate a particular speech sound with a particular animal or toy. This proves useful in evaluating listening skills. Children at this stage may not be able to cope with formal imitation exercises or assessment of perception of Ling's Five Sounds (oo, ah, ee, sh, ss – Ling, 1988) and, as clarified earlier, the early enforcement of repetition may not be productive. Perception of the Five Sounds can be assessed through play; observing the child's responses to 'sh' or 'ee' will enable even subtle changes in listening skills to be monitored.

Listening to speech sounds: developing discrimination at the transitional stage

Once the child has developed responses to a range of speech sounds, the development of discrimination is encouraged. The aim is to increase discrimination in the following areas:

- A single sound versus a repeated sound; e.g. a long train going 'choo, choo, choo' versus a short train going 'choo'.
- A long sound versus a short sound, e.g. a long snake going 'sssssssss' versus a short snake going 'ss'.

- A loud sound versus a quiet sound; e.g. a large sheep making a loud 'baa' versus a lamb with a quiet 'baa'.
- A high sound versus a low sound.
- One sound versus another, e.g. 'moo' versus 'baa'.

Games to promote the discrimination of speech sounds include the following activities on hearing the appropriate speech sound:

- Placing counters, or colouring, on an appropriate picture (see Figure 8.6 for examples).

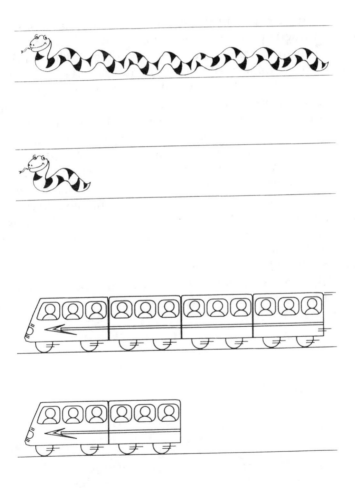

Figure 8.6 Examples of useful pictures for discriminating speech sounds: long versus short 'sss' and single versus repeated sound ('choo' versus 'choo choo choo'). The child colours, or places a counter, appropriately on hearing the sound

- Finding the appropriate hidden animal.
- Throwing a ball or hoop at toy animals.
- Racing animals (toy or puppet) along a track.
- Racing vehicles along a track, making different noises for each vehicle, as illustrated in Figure 8.7.
- Taking a pencil for a 'walk', varying the pattern in response to the sounds, for example, according to whether the stimulus was continous or repeated.
- Using a pencil or crayon to complete the path of a figure across a page, as in pre-writing left to right patterning activities, for example, moving the pram across the page in response to 'sh'.

Even young children can put counters on the long or short snakes according to whether the sound was long or short (Figure 8.6) or move a large or small animal along the track, according to whether the sound was loud or quiet. Initially all these tasks are carried out with the child able to lipread if he wishes; gradually opportunity must be taken in play to perform these games when the child is not in eye contact, so that the extent of developing listening skills may be assessed and reliance on audition promoted. Face-watching opportunities should be withdrawn in a natural way, rather than by covering the mouth with one's hand. Children become very adept at speechreading even when one's mouth is 'hidden'; they look intently for other facial clues, and in reality may not be dependent on audition. It is possible to carry out listening activities side by side, with the child focused on the book, paper, toy or activity while one is talking, ensuring the child is not lipreading, but listening in a natural, unforced manner. The child may attempt the sounds himself so that the adult can move the appropriate animal or vehicle. If the adult prefers to act the fool and make silly mistakes the child will love to correct these (proving, of course, that he is able to perform the task himself).

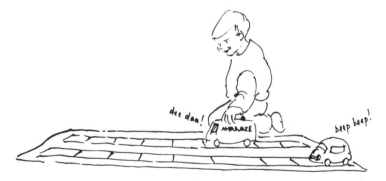

Figure 8.7 Race games encourage the discrimination of speech sounds; here the child listens and responds appropriately to 'dee daa' (ambulance) or 'beep beep' (car)

When the children are able to cooperate in the games described, and are able to demonstrate the ability to discriminate a range of speech sounds, they will usually be using some of these sounds in communication, have developed an understanding of the rules of communication and be equal partners in conversation. These children are at the functional language stage.

Working with children with functional spoken language

In the authors' programme, a small proportion of children have functional spoken language at implantation, but it is anticipated that most implanted children will achieve functional spoken language within the first 3 years following implantation (see Chapter 11). At this stage, the children are able orally to:

- initiate conversation
- comment
- respond to questioning
- question others
- joke
- contradict.

Communication and interaction at this stage become a great deal easier and some activities found useful in developing listening to environmental sounds, musical instruments and spoken language are described.

Listening to environmental sounds at the functional language level

Although the emphasis is on providing access to spoken language via the speech processor, children at all stages may respond first to environmental sounds and those with functional language will be able to record their own listening progress in a variety of ways. They may be able to use written language, or drawings, to record their listening experiences, completing their own checklists of sounds heard and sorting into groups those they can and cannot hear, and those they can identify. Children who have had no significant auditory input for a number of years need opportunities to explore and comment on these sounds in their environment to enable them to begin to adjust to their new hearing. They also need to know that it is acceptable to indicate what they cannot yet hear, or identify, and when there is no sound. Taped environmental sounds may give practice in learning to identify these new sounds, but care must be taken to introduce only a few items at a time.

Listening to musical instruments at the functional language level

The use of musical instruments can be developed further at this stage. They can be classified by the child into those he can or cannot hear, without the exercise being made at all stressful, or the child feeling under test. 'Sound' words may not have seemed very relevant previously and the use of musical instruments provides opportunity for discussion about the quality of sounds made and the introduction of appropriate vocabulary as words such as squeak, rattle, scrape begin to have an auditory meaning. An electric organ (Figure 8.8) or music synthesiser is useful with older children who may enjoy experimenting with the different sounds it produces, and children can learn to describe the sounds they can hear, as they become able to discriminate between loud/quiet, single/repeated sounds. The awareness of high/low discrimination seems a little more difficult for children, and children below the ages of 7 or 8 years may experience great difficulty with this concept, although an electric organ provides many opportunities for experiment.

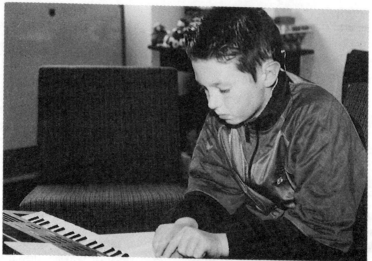

Figure 8.8 An electric organ provides opportunity to experiment with a variety of sounds

Older children enjoy using a personal stereo and listening to the usual 'pop' favourites; for a child who has missed out on peer group interests in pop music, this can be an important social experience too.

Listening to spoken language: the functional language level

Conversation

Once the child has developed some functional language the development of appropriate conversational skills is paramount. The most practical approach will often be to use the one-to-one conversation session in a quiet situation to develop listening skills in a natural way. As always, the child's interests can be the basis of the conversation, and the child's own contributions encouraged with the adult creating the context of the conversation. Topics could include home, family, pets, hobbies, television or comic characters; the important thing to remember is that the adult must talk *with* the child not *at* him (Webster and Wood, 1989), avoiding over-control by the adult. Before implantation, the child will have been unable to respond auditorally to spoken language; the child must now learn to use auditory clues, to take turn in conversation, to respond with appropriate eye contact as described with children at an earlier stage. The adult can facilitate this change in focus from visual modality to auditory modality by gradually withdrawing physical prompts and limiting distractions. The adult may need to continue to attract the child's attention visually to the conversation and its focus; gradually these extra cues must be reduced, so that the child becomes reliant on auditory prompts such as his name or the command 'listen' (Webster and Wood, 1989). For children in total communication settings, the rehabilitation programme should gradually extend the emphasis from sign to audition, as access to audition becomes possible. Auditory signals will become related to sign vocabulary over time (Tye-Murray, 1993); Tye-Murray gives useful guidelines for increasing the child's reliance on the auditory signal for communication.

The adult, as facilitator, bears some responsibility for ensuring that the listening environment for conversation is suitable for the child, particularly in the early stages following implantation, when listening in noise will be difficult. Background noise is difficult for cochlear implant wearers, as for hearing aid wearers, and classrooms should be acoustically treated to minimise reverberation, and parents be aware at home that background noise from the television, washing machine, running water and so on will affect their child's ability to listen (Tye-Murray, 1992). Immediately after implantation, conflicting noise may well hinder children's developing confidence in their listening abilities.

Opportunities must also be provided in class for small group conversation, and child–child interaction encouraged. Group conversation requires an appreciation of turn-taking at a higher level than on a one-to-one basis, and will provide the child with the experience of learning to follow the flow of conversation from one speaker to another with the conversation facilitated by an experienced listener.

Listening activities: spoken language

Discrimination of spoken language will be encouraged through the regular conversation sessions, but children at this stage still need some structured activities to develop reliance on audition and listening skills through the speech sound, word, phrase and sentence levels. Suggestions for activities to promote this development are now described; they must retain the element of fun and interaction which has already been emphasised and should be integrated into the child's everyday activities.

Figures with speech balloons into which the sound, word or phrase being given can be placed are adaptable for different children and are illustrated in Figure 8.9. Speech balloons containing Ling's Five Sounds can be used for children to indicate with counters or by ticking which sounds they are hearing. The speech balloons may show family names (beginning with those of differing numbers of syllables) as the child learns to discriminate one family name from another; if the child is unable to read then photographs are used. Finger puppets, or card pictures of faces talking to each other, provide opportunity to develop discrimination of words or phrases in an interactive setting.

Once the child has become able to discriminate single words, it is necessary to develop the discrimination of two- or three-word phrases,

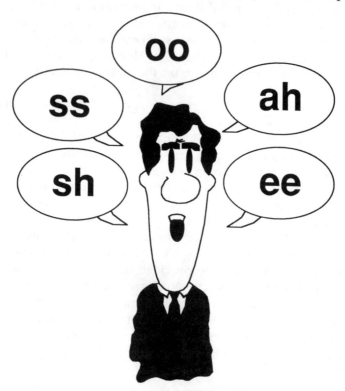

Figure 8.9 Speech balloons can be used to develop the discrimination of Ling's Five Sounds, names, single words, phrases or sentences; the child listens, and points or places a counter appropriately if unable to imitate

for example, hello Mummy versus bye-bye Mummy. Groups of pictures illustrating family members carrying out a variety of activities can be used to encourage discrimination of phrases; Mummy cooking: Mummy sleeping, for example. Card packs of various colour families are similiarly useful: Mummy Green in bed, Daddy Green in the car and so on are easily illustrated and the child learns to discriminate phrases by listening alone.

At the transitional stage cars and lorries were used, with the child and adult making speech sounds as they raced round the track. Once the child has functional language, it may be possible to use colours, numbers, days of the week, months of the year, figures using common phrases as listening tasks, incorporating the idea of a race into the activity. Race games previously used can easily be adapted to the child's interests using more complex language; favourite comic characters, vehicles, animals, puppets can race following oral instructions. In these games the teacher is able to provide opportunities for the child to develop listening further, and to observe the child's responses to spoken language as he moves different players in the game appropriately. The child is engrossed in the game, and the adult is able to use familiar, repetitive language, while retaining a high degree of motivation. Older children and those with functional language are able to cooperate with an adult or other children and will enjoy turn-taking games, thereby also acquiring valuable communication skills which may not have been learnt before implantation.

Activities that are appropriate to develop the discrimination of speech for children with functional language include the following:

- Races using oral instructions.
- Following oral instructions, for example, drawing or colouring a picture, making a model, carrying out a physical activity.
- Completing funny faces, figures or Mr Potato Head.
- Pelmanism (pick up pairs).
- Bingo/lotto, particularly if the child is asked to guess the card the adult is describing.
- Board games such as The House That Jack Built, Quack Quack.
- Memory games, for instance, lists can be given orally and each child repeats the list and adds another item of his choice.
- Battleships, using oral clues.
- Treasure hunts on a grid, given oral clues.
- Map-finding games, given oral clues.
- Guess who?
- Simon Says.
- Dot-to-Dot pictures completed orally.
- Guess what I'm thinking of? The adult describes a picture or article and the child names it or draws it.

Teachers of the deaf commonly use communication games with children to promote effective communication between children and adult–child, i.e. games in which children and teacher have to relay messages or instructions to each other effectively. Following implantation they are a useful way of giving the child a secure setting in which he can develop auditory skills. Conventional games such as Battleships, Guess who?, following instructions to find the treasure or one's way about a map, are all useful ways to motivate a child to wish to communicate. When trying to follow instructions on a map or grid, the difference between C1 and D1, for example, is very difficult to ascertain without listening and thus the child is placed in a non-threatening situation where he has to listen to be able to play the game. All these games can be useful means of involving other family members (Figure 8.10)

Development of listening through stories

Stories are an essential part of the child's learning to use sound in communication and have been found to play an important part in developing linguistic skills (Wells, 1981). Stories should have an amusing element – it helps both child and teacher to retain interest! Children enjoy personal contributions by their teachers, particularly if the teacher has done something they perceive as foolish; these personal stories can be illustrated and used as sequence stories for repeated telling and enacting. Comics are a fruitful source of amusing stories and adapting the current favourite character can be profitable. Comic stories can be cut up into picture sequence so that they can be sorted and re-told; the speech balloons can be blanked out so that the child

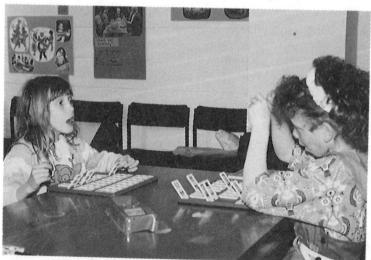

Figure 8.10 Communication games enable siblings and peers to be part of the rehabilitation programme

can complete the story in his own words. Several goals can be achieved in this way: in re-telling the story, the child can hear and experiment with different voices, learning to express a variety of feelings.

Children should have regular opportunity to hear a story and re-tell it, developing their own narrative skills with confidence. Familiar and repetitive stories and rhymes give opportunity to develop confidence in listening, and children enjoy listening for deliberate mistakes made by teacher or parent in the re-telling of a familiar story. Sequence stories in picture form are commonly used with deaf children and there are many sources of material. Once the pictures have been used to develop the story line, with the child predicting events, then they can be used as a listening activity in which the child is asked to identify the appropriate picture by listening for the corresponding sentence, thus developing listening skills at a higher level than the phrase level.

There are many story books available today with no text which are ideal for telling and re-telling stories. Traditional fairy tales contain many repetitive elements which again are ideal for children to re-tell or act out with their peers; those with finger puppets lend themselves to re-telling by child and parent or teacher in a variety of ways.

Development of listening through written language

With school-aged children the reinforcement that comes with using the written word is very helpful; it can be introduced gradually, with a great deal of repetition in stories about themselves. As with a hearing child, the most useful way of introducing the written word is through the child's own story books about himself. For example, different members of the family may be illustrated involved in a variety of activities at home. Each picture may have a simple phrase or sentence written underneath at the child's own linguistic level. The more amusing the activities, the better the chance of gaining and sustaining interest. Older children tell us that seeing the written pattern while hearing it is helpful in learning to listen to spoken language. The consistent visual pattern appears to reinforce the new auditory pattern if simple stories about themselves with picture clues are written for the child to follow visually on paper, while listening to the story being read by the adult. Stories containing four or five pictures are sufficient initially, and the use of speech balloons in the story encourage an interactive element. Shared reading reinforces the emphasis on meaningful interaction, and lack of adult control; sharing a book in this way provides an ideal means of assessing listening skills without putting the child in a 'test' situation (Figure 8.11). The focus of shared interest is naturally on the book and written word, and it is easy for the adult to assess the level of the child's understanding without lipreading.

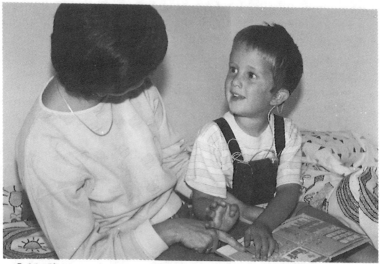

Figure 8.11 Sharing a book provides an ideal situation in which to learn to listen without lipreading when attention is on the book. Here the child has listened to his mother's contribution, interpreted it, and looks up to comment himself

Poems can also be useful, particularly amusing ones; they give the added clue of rhythm as the child attempts to follow the written script without lipreading. The adult may read and stop so that the child follows the written pattern and finds where the adult has paused. Amusing poems enable the teacher to use them several times for reinforcement, while retaining the child's interest and giving opportunity for shared enjoyment.

Connected Discourse Tracking (CDT – De Filippo and Scott, 1978) is an accepted procedure for adults which can usefully be adapted for children with functional spoken language. The adult reads the story in small phrases to the child, who then repeats each portion. If the child is unable to repeat, there are several recognised strategies: repeating, rephrasing, breaking down further, or using written or signed clues. The session is timed, usually about 5 minutes, and the number of words that the child has been able to repeat correctly per minute calculated. CDT is often used as a method of evaluation, with which there are many recognised difficulties (Tye-Murray and Tyler, 1988), but it can be a useful, meaningful, rehabilitation task. The authors have adapted the 'Mr Men' books (Hargreaves) for CDT: the child is able to see the picture but has to repeat the story, given initially with lipreading, then without. A series such as the 'Mr Men' books provide a wide variety of materials with the same format, and are of interest to children of a wide age range, making them very appropriate for repeated use with the same child.

Along with the use of the written form as an aid to rehabilitation, the authors have found a phonic approach to reading very helpful. While recognising the inherent problems in using a phonic approach with English and the fact that it emphasises a weakness for deaf children (Webster and Wood, 1989), it does give a child learning to use audition confidence and word attack skills. Early play with letters and initial sounds gives opportunity for repetition of speech sounds with an additional helpful visual input. It may also enable the child to achieve age-appropriate success with his class peers. Games such as 'I-Spy' can be played at home and school alike.

Many teachers of the deaf and therapists use computer-based activities in their work, and children with cochlear implants find these helpful too. Language programs and games with the child sitting side by side with the teacher at the computer give opportunity for conversation while the focus of visual attention is on the screen; this provides a natural situation in which there is the need to be reliant on audition. The use of a language tape-card machine, such as that in Figure 8.12, involves the child in using relevant written words and sentences, with opportunity for repeated listening and also for attempted repetition by the child.

Use of telephone

Many children find it very intimidating to use the telephone early in their use of the implant system and the best introduction is the way in which young hearing children first become accustomed to the

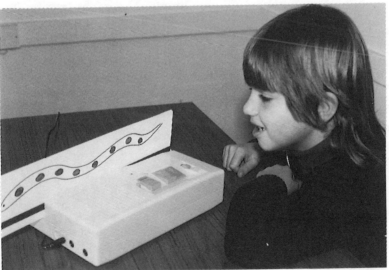

Figure 8.12 A language tape-card machine appropriate for use with young children; it gives practice in responding to, and discriminating, speech sounds and phrases. Here the child is listening to, and imitating, a long 'ssss'; it can, however, be used to develop discrimination of words, phrases and sentences

telephone, i.e. after a long period of confidence in spoken language to be encouraged to 'say hello to Daddy' (or any known adult), and to be allowed to do so over the telephone and to listen to the response and then say 'bye-bye'. The child can then become accustomed to the sound of the voice over the telephone in a known format and develop confidence in its use. Children who are tested over the telephone at this stage by an over-enthusiastic adult are often deterred by failure from further trials. Adult implant users report finding telephone training difficult, and children need sensitive handling in these early stages if they are to succeed.

A hearing child or an adult can be helpful in the beginning to encourage simple conversations, and children who can read find it very helpful to follow a simple script, which they have previously helped to write, over the telephone. The child and the adult on each end of the telephone each need a copy of the script, and read their part of the conversation. Once confidence has been built up in this way, children can then begin listening to simple 'tests' over the telephone: guessing who it is being named (from a limited set at first); guessing what the weather is like at the other end; guessing what the other person is eating or doing. Children with implants enjoy games listening to the telephone, but, like all children, they can be intimidated by it, and need to experience success in its use. The most powerful motivation will be when the child really needs to use the telephone to contact his parents or friends (Figure 8.13).

Conclusion

Teaching children to learn to interpret auditory signals is not new: many teachers have commented that following implantation the child is

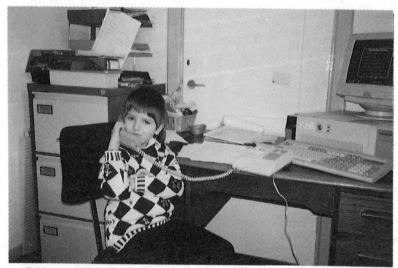

Figure 8.13 Learning to use the telephone

able to participate in many class activities which were previously inappropriate as they required some useful hearing. Children with cochlear implants may not require more rehabilitation time than those with hearing aids; rather it may be that the time spent with them after implantation will have a different focus and different expectations to those before implantation. It is becoming increasingly apparent that the true benefits of cochlear implantation only accrue over several years, particularly with young children. Over time, there are tremendous possibilities: those of us involved in paediatric cochlear implantation have a responsibility to ensure that the children in our care have the time and opportunities needed to use the new auditory signals being received to their full potential.

Acknowledgements

The authors are grateful to Maureen Copley for the illustrations, and to colleagues and Amy Robbins of Indiana University School of Medicine for comments on earlier drafts of this chapter.

References

Boothroyd, A. (1989). Hearing aids, cochlear implants and profoundly deaf children. In E. Owens and D.K. Kessler (eds), *Cochlear Implants in Young Deaf Children*. Boston: Little, Brown & Co.

Boothroyd, A. (1991). Assessment of speech perception capacity in profoundly deaf children. *American Journal of Otology*, **12**, 67–72.

Bruner, J.S. (1983). *Child's Talk: Learning to Use Language*. Oxford: Oxford University Press.

Cooper, H. (1991). Training and rehabilitation for cochlear implant users. In H. Cooper (ed.), *Cochlear Implants: A Practical Guide*. London: Whurr.

De Filippo, C.L. and Scott, B.L. (1978). A method for training and evaluating the reception of ongoing speech. *Journal of the Accoustical Society of America*, **63**, 1186–1192.

Eisenberg, L.S. (1985). Perceptual capabilities with the cochlear implant: Implications for aural rehabilitation. *Ear and Hearing*, **6** (3), 60S–69S.

Fryauf-Bertschy, H. (1992). Getting started at home. In N. Tye-Murray (ed.), *Cochlear Implants and Children: A Handbook for Parents and Teachers and Speech And Hearing Professionals*. Washington DC: Alexander Graham Bell Association for the Deaf.

Gross, H. (1987). Social interaction and play in the deaf nursery school. Unpublished PhD Thesis, University of Nottingham.

Hargreaves, R. *The Mr Men Series*. London: Thurman Publishing.

Ling, D. (1988). *Foundations of Spoken Language for Hearing Impaired Children*. Washington DC: Alexander Graham Bell Association for the Deaf.

McCormick, B. (1991). Paediatric cochlear implantation in the UK – a delayed journey along a well marked route. *British Journal of Audiology*, **25**, 145–149.

Osberger, M.J. (1990). Audiological rehabilitation with cochlear implants and tactile aids. *Asha*, **32**, 38–43.

Somers, M. (1991). Speech perception abilities in children with cochlear implants and hearing aids. *American Journal of Otology*, **12**, 174–178.

Tait, M. (1984). The role of singing in the social and linguistic development of nursery aged deaf children. Unpublished PhD Thesis, University of Nottingham.

Tait, M. (1987). Making and monitoring progress in the pre-school years. *Journal of the British Association of Teachers of the Deaf*, **11** (5), 143.

Tye-Murray, N. (ed.) (1992). *Cochlear Implants and Children: A Handbook for Parents, Teachers and Speech and Hearing Professionals*. Washington DC: Alexander Graham Bell Association for the Deaf.

Tye-Murray, N. (1993). Aural rehabilitation and patient management. In R.S. Tyler (ed.), *Cochlear Implants: Audiological Foundations*. San Diego, CA: Singular.

Tye-Murray, N. and Tyler, R.A. (1988). A critique of continuous discourse tacking as a text procedure. *Journal of Speech and Hearing Disorders*, **53**, 226–231.

Webster, A. (1992). Images of deaf children as learners. In T. Cline (ed.), *The Assessment of Special Educational Needs: International Perspectives*. London: Routledge.

Webster, A. and Wood, D. (1989). *Special Needs in Ordinary Schools: Children with Hearing Difficulties*. London: Cassell.

Wells, G. (1981). *Learning Through Interaction*. Cambridge: Cambridge University Press.

Wood, D.J., Wood, H.A., Griffith, A.J. and Howarth, C.I. (1986). *Teaching and Talking With Deaf Children*. London: John Wiley.

Chapter 9
Monitoring progress in children at the pre-verbal stage

SUE ARCHBOLD

Evaluating the potential changes in communication and spoken language skills, educational achievements, and social and emotional development which may be brought about by cochlear implantation is a vital part of the work of an implant programme. This chapter looks briefly at some of the problems in assessing changes in young deaf children with little spoken language. It then describes one particular measure, a profile of listening skills, which is being developed by the Nottingham programme and has been found to be useful for monitoring the acquisition of listening skills in young children in the first year following implantation.

The difficulties in assessing progress in young deaf children are well recognised (Boothroyd, 1991; Osberger et al., 1991a; Staller et al., 1991a): the lack of homogeneity in the group, difficulties controlling for aetiology, age of onset, maturation and educational management. These difficulties led the trials of the Food and Drug Administration (FDA) of the Nucleus 22 channel system to use a single-subject, repeated-measures design (Mecklenburg, Demorest and Staller, 1991). In addition, the interactions among these factors make the isolation of variables that might predict benefit problematic. For example, children with later onset of deafness are more likely to be in oral educational settings than those with early onset (Osberger, 1990).

Assessing the benefit received by children fitted with Nucleus 22 channel cochlear implants has largely been seen in terms of measuring changes in speech perception and production after implantation (Osberger et al., 1991b; Staller et al., 1991b; Osberger, Maso and Sam, 1993). The most rapidly growing group of implantees, however, is the age group 2–4 years, comprising children who may have little or no spoken language, and few of the communication skills that form the precursors of speech and language development.

There are few measures available for such children who are often unable to carry out the simplest imitative task (Beiter, Staller and Dowell, 1991; Osberger et al., 1991a); tests that are available have problems of low test/re-test reliability, mode of presentation, vocabulary and number of test items, all of which may influence the evaluation (Osberger et al., 1991a). Boothroyd (1991) and Tyler (1993) discuss the difficulties in developing tests of speech perception for young deaf children. Tyler emphasises the need for tests to be within the language and vocabulary capabilities of the child, their cognitive and motor abilities and attention span. As Dyar stresses in Chapter 11, assessments made of these children must assess what is assessable.

Tests of perception described as being appropriate for young children with cochlear implants include the Discrimination after Training (DAT) test (Thielemeir,1984) and the low-verbal version of the Early Speech Perception Test (Geers and Moog, 1987), both of which demand some linguistic ability. The Aided Articulation Index (Gittleman and Popelka, 1987), based on aided and unaided thresholds, has been used by some to predict speech perception ability, but has not been validated on children with cochlear implants (Geers and Moog, 1989). Geers and Moog (1987) categorised the speech perception abilities of deaf children into four groups: no pattern perception, pattern perception, some word recognition and consistent word recognition. This categorisation has been used to show changes over time with implanted children, but is not sensitive enough to mark progress in young children in the early stages following implantation. The Listening Skills Development Sequence of Somers (1991) is useful in giving a guide to the identification of changes in listening skills, but it does not provide quantifiable outcomes.

The purpose of assessment

In spite of the difficulties in designing appropriate tests, with reported wide variation in individual outcomes following implantation, it is vital that paediatric implant teams develop a sensitive and appropriate assessment battery for all children in their care, however young (see also Chapters 10 and 11). The principal aim of implantation is to give auditory access to speech that was not possible with conventional hearing aids. The progress of each child must be monitored in use of audition from the very earliest stages following implantation to assess benefit, monitor tuning and functioning of the device, and to evaluate the effectiveness of the rehabilitation programme (Boothroyd, 1991). With growing evidence of intermittent faults with hardware (Tyler and Kelsay, 1990), which can be difficult to identify in children with little language to describe what they hear, and the complexity of device tuning in children unable to comment on sound quality, it is essential that regular assessments of progress are made. These enable the child's use of the device to be monitored and promote optimal functioning of the device at all times. In addition, in future, it will become increasingly important to assess the relative benefits of different devices for children.

In addition to monitoring individual progress for clinical purposes, outcome measures are needed to respond to the many questions being asked about implantation. There is little consensus on criteria for selection of candidates who are likely to do well after implantation (Osberger, 1990) or on the most effective forms of rehabilitation (Cooper, 1991). Obtaining rigorous outcome measures over time should enable more rational decisions to be made on appropriate candidature and effective management. The controversy which continues to surround paediatric implantation can best be resolved by careful and objective documentation of progress and problems. In times of increasing financial accountability and scrutiny in health care services throughout the world, benefits arising from paediatric implantation must be quantified by consistent collection of outcome data on every implanted child (O'Donoghue, 1992).

The role of parents and educators in assessment

This book has emphasised the role of parents and of the child's own teacher of the deaf following implantation. Vidas, Hassan and Parnes (1992) found that clinical tests of speech and hearing may not reflect the child's performance at home and school and, like Selmi (1985) and Cunningham (1990), that the perceptions reported by parents, teachers and clinic therapists differ widely. Cunningham (1990) found that parents considered that their child performed significantly better in structured (training) situations than in unstructured (real-life) situations. To document performance outside the clinic they suggested that assessments should involve parents and teachers. Monitoring progress in real life as well as in a clinical test situation gives a more comprehensive picture of a child's functioning; a great deal of research into children's learning has moved from clinical testing to observation at home and school for this reason (Webster and Wood, 1989). If it is to be possible for the implant team to monitor progress in everyday situations, as well as in the clinic, then the child's parents and educators must be actively involved in the process.

There is a danger that teachers may feel suspicious of researchers who arrive in the classroom seemingly to gather data to confirm their own hypotheses, and feel that the ensuing research reports may not accurately reflect the reality of the situation. Wood (1981) expresses the difficulty of an external researcher in understanding the teacher's aims, underlying philosophy and classroom practice, and stresses the need for an external researcher to work cooperatively, using the teacher's expertise and insights. A member of the implant team, in entering the local teacher's domain, is rather like the external researcher, and must develop ways of using the insights of the child's teacher to gain a full picture of the child's functioning.

For the reasons outlined above, the Nottingham Paediatric Cochlear Implant Programme is developing and refining a battery of assessments for use with young children, who function at the pre-verbal stage. The battery includes video analyses, questionnaires for parents, teachers and therapists, and skilled observations and profiles. Standardised tests are also used as these become appropriate. These assessments measure changes in the following areas:

- Use of the implant system and adaptation to it
- Environmental sound detection and recognition
- Early communication skills
- Development of speech reception skills
- Development of speech production
- Linguistic development
- Social skills/independence/behaviour
- Parental expectations and attitudes.

Chapter 10 describes one well-established measure based on video analysis. This chapter now outlines the rationale and development of a profile designed to assess listening skills in young pre-verbal children in the first year following implantation, termed 'listening progress' (LiP). The use of LiP and the results obtained with the first 18 young children in the Nottingham programme are then discussed. Throughout, the teacher of the deaf working at the implant clinic will be referred to as the *implant clinic teacher*, and the child's teacher of the deaf as *the local teacher*.

Listening progress (a profile to assess the developing use of audition in pre-verbal cochlear implant users)

Rationale

Aided sound field audiometry gives a measure of sensitivity – the ability to detect the auditory signal through the implant – but there is also a need to measure the child's developing ability to listen to and interpret the signal. A child who is audiologically suitable for implantation will generally have been unable to respond to spoken language presented auditorally in conversational situations. The pattern of social interaction in which the child develops pre-verbal skills, such as turn-taking,

discussed in Chapter 10, may have been disrupted. Following implantation, he or she should be able to respond to auditory stimuli within the
familiar, repetitive settings found to promote linguistic skills. The
Nottingham team places much emphasis on the use of the game formats described in Chapter 8, which have been found to promote verbal
interaction in a way that would have been inappropriate or unsuccess-
ful before implantation, without access to spoken language through
audition. Attempts to monitor progress by enforced repetition of specific speech sounds disrupts the normal patterns of adult–child interaction and may not give an accurate representation of the child's
progress.

Test development and construction

Listening progress was developed as part of the Nottingham programme's assessment battery as a profile for the development of early
listening skills, including environmental as well as speech sounds. It
does not place the child in a 'test' situation, but gathers information by
proxy about the child's developing listening abilities within normal
rehabilitation settings in home and school. Although emphasis is put
on the adult's appropriate response to the child's contributions, the
rehabilitation activities at Nottingham have an underlying structure in
which the *implant clinic teacher* maintains an overview of the probable sequential development of listening skills. Erber's (1982) hierarchical listening categories of detection, discrimination, identification and
comprehension are commonly used in describing listening progress;
LiP covers the early stages of detection (response), discrimination and
the first stages of identification.

The development of LiP was influenced by several factors:

- Discussions with other implant teams, and knowledge of the literature which identified the shortage of such appropriate tests for pre-
  verbal children.
- The need for an assessment of listening skills with activities appropriate to the age, interest, and linguistic and cognitive abilities of the
  child.
- The need for an assessment which involved the participation of the
  child in settings which closely resembled real-life situations.
- The need to describe progress or otherwise in listening skills in
  young children to parents and professionals.

Additionally, the construction of the profile was influenced by other
factors:

- The consistent format of regular reports made by *implant clinic
  teachers* following rehabilitation sessions.

- The need for information on children's listening progress to be clearly set out and accessible to a variety of individuals.
- The development in the UK of the Department of Health evaluation of paediatric implantation, and the requirement to document progress in these young children by methods suitable for qualitative analysis on large groups of implanted children.

The record sheet for LiP is illustrated in Figure 9.1. Initial responses to (detection of) environmental and speech sounds are scored, with differentiation between those that are spontaneous and those that are elicited. It is often possible to elicit a response to a sound in a game before the child will respond spontaneously. Increasing ability to dis-

	Pre	Post	3mth	6mth	12mth	24mth	36mth
Response to environmental sounds							
Response to drum (elicited)							
Response to musical instruments (elicited)							
Response to voice - elicited							
spontaneous							
Discrimination between two musical instruments							
Discrimination between: Loud/quiet drum							
single/repeated drum							
Identification of environmental sounds							
Response to: /oo/							
/ah/							
/ee/							
/sh/							
/ss/							
Discrimination between: Long/short speech sounds							
single/repeated speech sounds							
loud/quiet speech sounds							
two of Ling's five sounds							
all of Ling's five sounds							
Discrimination between two family names of different syllabic length							
Identification of own name in quiet							
Totals:							

Always (2); Sometimes (1); Never/Not Known (0)

Figure 9.1 Listening progress (LiP): record sheet

criminate one sound from another and progress towards ability to identify sounds in isolation is observed, with the maximum score being obtained when the child is able to identify his or her own name (without lipreading) in quiet surroundings at home and at school; beyond this stage more conventional measures can be taken. The measure includes response to, and increasing discrimination of, Ling's Five Sounds (Ling, 1988). This procedure is regularly used by implant teams as a check on device functioning. It should be noted that the record sheet is not hierarchical, for example, response to speech sounds will be observed before identification of environmental sounds.

Responses are scored Always (A), Sometimes (S), and Never/Not Known (N); the Appendix gives the scoring procedures with the required behaviour and acceptable response. Each Never/Not Known response is scored as zero; each response of Sometimes is scored as one and each Always response is scored as two; the total score is then calculated. The assessment is carried out by an *implant clinic teacher* and is discussed fully with the child's parents and *local teacher* to ensure that scores reflect as accurately as possible the child's use of the implant system at home and at school. Any discrepancies in scoring are discussed. Each child is assessed before implantation, immediately after the first fitting of the device and at 3, 6, 12 and 24 months following initial tuning.

Subjects

Listening progress is used with all the children in the author's programme and results are given here for the first 18 children with early onset of deafness, before the age of 3 years. Before implantation all children had aided thresholds 70 dB(A) across the frequency range 500 Hz to 4 kHz, when wearing appropriate aids with good earmoulds and no middle-ear complications.

Table 9.1 shows the age of onset of hearing loss, age at implantation, length of deafness in years and educational communication management (oral/aural, OA, or total communication, TC) of these children. This analysis emphasises individual differences between children, rather than representing only group data.

Three of the children were congenitally deaf (020, 021, 027); all the others were deafened by meningitis, apart from 006. At the time of implantation the mean duration of deafness was 3.3 years and the mean age of onset was 1.3 years. The children were placed in the variety of educational settings to be found within the UK: schools for the deaf, units for the deaf within mainstream schools, mainstream schools and at the pre-school level. Oral/aural and total communication systems may be found within any of these settings; ten of the children were in oral settings and eight were using total communication.

Table 9.1 Background information on the subjects

CIN*	Age at onset (years)	Age at implant (years)	Length of deafness (years)	Communication management†
002	2.1	5.0	2.9	OA
003	2.7	3.5	0.8	OA
004	2.7	6.5	3.8	OA
005	2.0	8.4	6.4	TC
006	1.2	2.7	1.5	TC
010	0.6	4.1	3.5	TC
011	2.8	3.6	0.8	OA
012	1.0	2.5	1.5	OA
013	1.1	2.8	1.7	OA
014	0.7	3.6	3.0	OA
016	2.1	7.3	5.2	TC
017	0.7	4.3	3.6	TC
018	2.6	8.6	6.0	OA
020	0.0	4.4	4.4	OA
021	0.0	3.4	3.4	TC
023	0.6	5.1	4.5	TC
024	0.8	2.9	2.1	OA
027	0.0	3.5	3.5	TC
Mean	**1.3**	**4.6**	**3.3**	

*CIN is the child's case number.
†OA is oral/aural educational setting; TC is total communication setting.

Results

Reliability of Listening progress (LiP)

Although the emphasis during rehabilitation is on following the child's interests, the *implant clinic teacher* influences the activities chosen so that the profile is repeatable across children and by different users. Following the development of LiP by the first two teachers of the deaf to be appointed in Nottingham, the arrival of a third teacher gave the opportunity to ensure that the scoring of responses was consistent and clarify any ambiguities in the scoring procedures (see Appendix). Further checks on the reliability of the measure were made when each of the three *implant clinic teachers* asked three *local teachers* to carry out the profile independently for the child. In this way, the scores for nine children at different intervals were cross-checked, and the results of the implant clinic teachers were compared with the local teachers. The scores are compared in Figure 9.2; the high repeatability is demonstrated by the high correlation coefficient relating the replicates ($r = 0.969$).

The large measure of agreement between the children's *local teachers*, who work with them daily, and their *implant clinic teachers* indicates that LiP is repeatable, and hence reliable. The child's *local teacher*

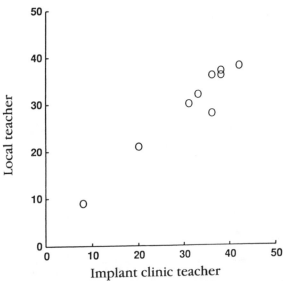

Figure 9.2 Replications of LiP scores (max. A2): the results for nine children, comparing the scores of the *local teachers* with the *implant clinic teachers*, at the same intervals

and the *implant clinic teacher* in the Nottingham programme have very similar perceptions of the child's listening abilities, unlike those in the study by Vidas, Hassan and Parnes (1992). Whether this is the result of LiP giving a more accurate reflection of the child's listening abilities in real life, or whether the closeness of the scores is influenced by the large degree of cooperative work carried out by the implant clinic and local teachers, is not clear and requires further investigation.

In only one case was there a material difference in scores; in that case the child functioned very differently at home and at school. His educational setting strongly emphasised the use of sign language, with low expectations of audition. At home, and in sessions with the *implant clinic teacher*, the child chose to use an oral mode of communication, and demonstrated good use of developing listening skills which were not observed in school. In addition, the child's result on the Meaningful Auditory Integration Scale (MAIS – Robbins, 1990) was very much lower when completed by his teacher at school than when it was completed by his parents, showing much less evidence of attaching meaning to sound in school than at home.

Progress of children over time using LiP

The mean scores for the group are given in Figure 9.3 as a function of time. The mean score for the group before implantation was 1%, whereas the mean score 1 year later was 89%. The only observed pre-operative response for any of the children was that elicited to a loud

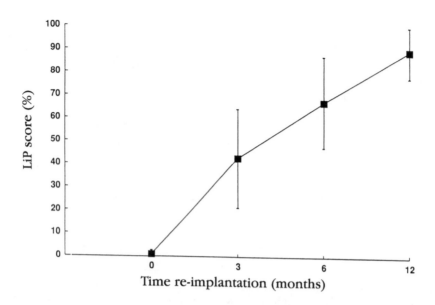

Figure 9.3 Listening progress (LiP): mean scores (%) during the first year after implantation for 18 young children with early onset of deafness. The error bars indicate ± 1 standard deviation and have been truncated at 0% and 100%

drum and only one child (013) showed some awareness of environmental sounds before implantation. Staller et al. (1991b) comment on the high intersubject variability with children. Although the group means show a steady increase over time, the size of the standard deviation in this group also indicates large intersubject variability, making it important to look at individual data. Table 9.2 gives the individual scores of the children at each assessment interval.

Looking at the measures over time, all children showed general and highly significant positive changes in the growth of listening skills based on a repeated-measures analysis of variance ($p<0.0001$). There were no children who showed a decrease in score at successive evaluation points, and only one child's score (018) remained the same at successive evaluation points. Greatest changes in score are seen in the first 3 months after implantation, as is also shown by video analysis (Chapter 10) of vocal turn-taking. Vocal turn-taking involves the development of early communication skills; in the early stages LiP demands only response to a range of sounds, and the changes in score in the first 3 months mark subtle changes in listening skills. All children, however, continue to show increases in listening progress scores throughout the first 12 months after implantation; 5 of the 18 children had reached the maximum score after 1 year.

The two children for whom progress was slowest (010 and 012)

Table 9.2 LiP scores during the first year after implantation for 18 children with early onset of deafness

CIN	Pre-implant score (%)	Score (%) measured after implantation		
		3 months	6 months	12 months
002	2	71	86	98
003	2	29	88	100
004	0	14	38	83
005	2	90	95	100
006	2	29	56	95
010	0	31	43	69
011	0	52	93	100
012	0	7	24	64
013	7	24	57	100
014	0	33	76	93
016	2	56	71	90
017	0	31	71	95
018	2	76	76	90
020	0	52	76	100
021	0	48	74	86
023	0	45	79	81
024	0	36	57	95
027	0	43	48	71
Mean scores	1	43	67	89

CIN is child's case number

were both children for whom it was difficult to obtain accurate measurements of maximum comfort levels, and therefore achieve optimum processor settings, in tuning sessions in the first year. Two years after implantation it was found that 010 had a faulty electrode which may have been causing her some difficulty in auditory discrimination earlier. Both these children had attained the maximum score by the 2-year evaluation point. Only one child (004) did not attain the maximum score by the 2-year evaluation point and is considered further below.

Discussion of the use of LiP

One of the aims of LiP was to monitor the functioning and tuning of the device. This has been borne out in practice, and LiP has helped to identify intermittent faults with processors, for example, when a child had been found to be unable to carry out a listening task previously within his capabilities. The complex tuning of the Nucleus system can be difficult to accomplish with young children, and reports of progress or problems in the developing use of audition are useful to those responsible for tuning. In one instance, for example, the fact that the child was reported to be unable to respond to /sss/ helped to identify more quickly a required change in tuning at the next clinic visit. On other occasions, LiP helped to identify other problems either with the child or the system of management. One child (004) was making progress in auditory processing, as demonstrated by LiP, but was not showing gains on other measures involving the use of language. The measurement of subtle steps in auditory processing using LiP, plus the demonstration of appropriate aided sound field response levels, good vocal turn-taking skills (see Chapter 10), good adaptation to the device, as measured by the MAIS (Robbins, 1990), and good environmental sound identification confirmed adequate auditory function. This led the author's group to look elsewhere for the cause of the child's inability to acquire spoken language. The use of Osberger et al.'s (1991b) video analysis of spontaneous speech also revealed, at the 6-month stage, that the child was not demonstrating the ability to encode speech. Further investigation by a clinical psychologist and the team speech and language therapist identified the existence of a specific language learning problem, which may well have been an additional consequence of meningitis. This was not identifiable before the acquisition of useful hearing through the implant.

An important use for LiP, which was not foreseen, was the evidence it gave parents and teachers of the efficacy of the device. This was particularly so in the early stages following implantation, when the signs of progress may be subtle. Parents find these early stages stressful (Quittner et al., 1991), and teachers may feel frustrated and unconvinced about the efficacy of the device when there may be little obvious evidence of progress (Osberger et al., 1991c). The demonstration and identification of small progressive steps in learning to listen can encourage parents and teachers, largely responsible for the day-to-day management of the child, to have realistic expectations of audition and to persevere in the use of the system.

Continuing work on LiP

Work is continuing to compare LiP with other measures such as video analysis (see Chapter 10; Osberger et al., 1991b) and to document influences on progress. These influences include those that are outside the control of the implant programme, such as age of onset and length of deafness, and those that are potentially open to manipulation, such as management style and communication style. Other questions which remain to be answered are whether early good progress in listening as measured by LiP is a predictor of later use of audition and development of language and other skills. The continued gathering of longitudinal data on these children will enable such questions to be addressed in the future.

More objective methods of implementing the profile are being considered including computer-based measures to overcome problems of live-voice presentation and repeatability. Children as young as 3 years (Boothroyd, 1991) are found to be able to cooperate with computer-based speech activities. Any developments, however, must be capable of being used in home and school, so that as the profile is refined it does not become a clinic-based tool.

General discussion

Paediatric cochlear implant programmes have a responsibility to monitor progress in the use of the implant system in all children in their care, including those with little or no language. For the reasons outlined earlier in this chapter, these are children for whom it will be difficult to monitor device functioning, or the appropriateness of the tuning strategy and rehabilitation programme by formal means. There remains, however, a shortage of appropriate tests, and, as Boothroyd (1991) states, 'the search continues' for those suitable for pre-verbal children. The indications are that LiP will prove one such tool. It is well suited to monitoring the development of the use of audition in these children, particularly in the first year after implantation, when more formal evidence of progress may be slight. It is vital that the battery of tests used by implant programmes include those suitable for the pre-verbal group, and that they include contributions by parents and teachers, so that as full a picture as possible of the child's functioning is obtained.

Acknowledgements

The author gratefully acknowledges the work of her colleagues in the development of LiP, and the constructive comments given by Professor Mary Joe Osberger of Indiana University School of Medicine, and Dr M.E. Lutman of the Institute of Hearing Research, Nottingham.

Appendix: Listening progress (LiP): notes for completion

Listening progress (LiP) is a profile of developing listening skills, completed by the implant clinic teacher of the deaf, using activities designed to elicit appropriate responses as part of the rehabilitation programme. Observations carried out during the rehabilitation programme, not necessarily a specific 'test' situation, will be accepted. The skills must be observed without lipreading or visual clue. (See our rehabilitation book for ideas for suitable games.)

The word 'response' is used to describe the detection of sound; 'discrimination' is used to describe the ability to choose correctly between two differing sounds; 'identification' to describe the ability to choose correctly the target sound from the open set of sounds. The child's performance may be scored:

N   (never/not known) if the skill has never been observed (0 points)
S   (sometimes) if the skill is becoming established and has been observed by the implant clinic teacher of the deaf at least once, but not consistently (1 point)
A   (always) if the skill is reported to be well established and the implant clinic teacher of the deaf has observed it consistently in more than two situations (2 points)

Behaviour/skills	Accepted response
Response to environmental sounds	Any awareness of environmental sounds shown, by spontaneous behavioural response
Response to drum (elicited)	A behavioural response to loud drum; elicited in play format (e.g. emerging from playhouse on sound of drum)
Response to musical instruments (elicited)	A behavioural response to at least two different musical instruments – maracas, bells, tambourine etc. (e.g. child rolls ball at skittles in response to sound)
Response to voice (elicited)	The child can perform a task on the spoken signal, for example, 'go' or 'boo' with voice at conversational sound level
Response to voice (spontaneous)	Reactions to voice in stories, singing, games formats, have been observed
Discrimination between two different instruments	The ability to discriminate (without being able to watch when the sound is made) between two differing musical instruments
Discrimination between loud/quiet drum	The ability to discriminate between loud and quiet drums, for example, by pointing to appropriate picture, or imitating sound
Discrimination between single/repeated drum	Again, pictures may be used to denote a drum being played once, or several times, and the child indicates by pointing at the picture. Alternatively, the child may be given a drum of his or her own and imitate the sound being made by the teacher out of sight

9	Identification of environmental sounds	Score S if the child is reported as identifying some environmental sounds at home/school and the implant clinic teacher of the deaf has observed the child identifying by sound alone at least one environmental sound. Score A if the implant clinic teacher of the deaf has observed the child identifying a range of environmental sounds at home/school and the child is monitoring his or her environment auditorily
10	Response to Ling's five sounds (/oo/, /ah/, /ee/, /sh/, /ss/)	The implant clinic teacher of the deaf, in a variety of game formats, observes the child's detection of the five sounds. For example, does the child move the sleeping baby on the sound /sh/. Score S if the skill is becoming established; score A if the child has been observed to carry out the tasks consistently
11	Discrimination between long/short speech sounds	The child can discriminate, for example, between a long /ba/ and a short /ba/ or a long /ss/ and a short /ss/ in a game
12	Single and repeated speech sounds	The child can discriminate, for example, between 'choo choo choo choo' (a long train) and 'choo' (a short train)
13	Loud and quiet speech sounds	The child can discriminate, for example, between the large toy dog giving a loud 'woof woof' and the toy puppy giving a quiet 'woof woof'
14	Discrimination between two of Ling's five sounds. For example, /oo/ versus /ee/, /sh/ versus /ss/	Score S if the child can discriminate between at least one combination of two of Ling's five sounds. Score A if the child can discriminate between any combination of two of Ling's five sounds
15	All of Ling's five sounds	Score S if the child is becoming able to identify any one sound out of the five; score A if the child is consistently able to identify all five sounds
16	Discrimination between two family names of differing syllabic length	Using family pictures, written names or the people themselves, can the child discriminate between two names of differing syllabic length, e.g. John versus Mummy
	Identification of own name	Score S if the child has been observed to identify his or her own name at home and school on at least one occasion; score A if the child can identify his or her own name (in reasonable listening conditions) consistently

References

Beiter, A.L., Staller, S.J. and Dowell, R.C. (1991). Evaluation and device programming in children. *Ear and Hearing,* **12** (4), 25S–33S.

Boothroyd, A. (1991). The assessment of speech perception capacity in profoundly deaf children. *American Journal of Otology,* **12** (Suppl.), 67–72.

Cooper, H. (1991). Training and rehabilitation for cochlear implant users. In H. Cooper (ed.), *Cochlear Implants: A Practical Guide* pp. 219–239. London: Whurr.

Cunningham, J.K. (1990). Parents' evaluation of the effects of 3M/House cochlear implants in children. *Ear and Hearing,* **11**, 375–381.

Erber, N.P. (1982). *Auditory Training.* Washington DC: Alexander Graham Bell Association for the Deaf.

Geers, A.E. and Moog, J.S. (1987). Predicting spoken language acquisition of profoundly hearing impaired children. *Journal of Speech and Hearing Disorders,* **52**, 84–94.

Geers, A.E. and Moog, J.S. (1989). Evaluating speech perception skills. In: Owens, E. and Kessler, D.K. (eds), *Cochlear Implant in Young Deaf Children*, pp. 227–256. Boston: Little & Brown.

Gittleman, D. and Popelka, G. (1987). The dynamic range configuration audiogram. *Volta Review,* **89**, 69–83.

Ling, D. (1988). *Foundations of Spoken Language for Hearing Impaired Children.* Washington DC: Alexander Graham Bell Association for the Deaf.

Mecklenberg, D.J., Demorest, M.E. and Staller, S.J. (1991). Scope and design of the clinical trial of the Nucleus multichannel cochlear implant in children. *Ear and Hearing,* **12** (4), 10S–14S.

O'Donoghue, G.M. (1992). Cochlear implants in children. *Journal of the Royal Society of Medicine,* **85**, 655–657.

Osberger, M.J. (1990). Audiological rehabilitation with cochlear implants and tactile aids. *Asha,* **32**, 38–43.

Osberger, M.J., Maso, M. and Sam, L.K. (1993). Speech intelligibility of children with cochlear implants, tactile aids or hearing aids. *Journal of Speech and Hearing Research,* **36**, 186–203.

Osberger, M.J., Miyamoto, R.T., Zimmerman-Phillips, S., Kemink, J.L., Stroer, B.S., Firszt, J.B. and Novak, M.A. (1991a). Independent evaluation of the speech perception abilities of children with the Nucleus 22 channel cochlear implant system. *Ear and Hearing,* **12** (4), 66S–80S.

Osberger, M.J., Robbins, A.M. Berry, S.W., Todd, S.L., Hesketh, L.J. and Sedey, A. (1991b). Analysis of the spontaneous speech samples of children with cochlear implants or tactile aids. *American Journal of Otology,* **12**, 151–164.

Osberger, M.J., Dettman, S.J., Daniel, K.C., Moog, J.S., Siebert, R., Stone, P. and Jorgensen, S. (1991c). Rehabilitation and education issues with implanted children: perspectives from a panel of clinicians and educators. *American Journal of Otology,* **12**, 205–212.

Quittner, A.L., Thompson, Steck, J. and Rouiller, R.L. (1991). Cochlear implants in children in study of parental stress and adjustment. *American Journal of Otology,* **12** (Suppl.), 95–104.

Robbins, A. (1990). Developing meaningful auditory integration in children with cochlear implants. *Volta Review,* **92**, 361–370.

Selmi, A. (1985). Monitoring and evaluating the educational effects of the cochlear implant. *Ear and Hearing,* **6** (3), 52S–59S.

- Somers, M.N. (1991). Effects of cochlear implants in children: Implications for rehabilitation. In H. Cooper (ed.), *Cochlear Implants: A Practical Guide*, pp. 322–345. London: Whurr.

- Staller, S.J., Beiter, A.L., Brimacombe, J.A., Mecklenburg, D.J. and Arndt, P. (1991a). Pediatric performance with the Nucleus 22 channel cochlear implant system. *American Journal of Otology*, **12**, 126–136.

- Staller, S.J., Dowell, R.C., Beiter, A.L. and Brimacombe, J.A. (1991b). Perceptual abilities of children with the Nucleus 22 channel cochlear implant. *Ear and Hearing*, **12**(4), 345–475.

Thielemeir, M.A. (1984). *Discrimination after Training*. Los Angeles: House Ear Institute.

Tyler, R.S. (1993). Speech perception by children. In R.S. Tyler (ed.), *Cochlear Implants: Audiological Foundations*, pp. 191–256. San Diego, CA: Singular.

Tyler, R.S. and Kelsay, D. (1990). Advantages and disadvantages reported by some of the better cochlear implant patients. *American Journal of Otology*, **11**, 282–289.

Vidas, S., Hassan, R. and Parnes, L.S. (1992). Real-life performance considerations of four pediatric multi-channel cochlear implant recipients. *Journal of Otolaryngology*, **21**, 387–393.

Webster, A. and Wood, D (1989). *Special Needs in Ordinary Schools: Children with Hearing Difficulties*. London: Cassell.

Wood, D.J. (1981). Theory and research in classrooms: lessons from deaf education. In W. Swan (ed.), *The Practice of Special Education*. Milton Keynes: Open University Press.

Chapter 10
Using video analysis to monitor progress in young cochlear implant users

MARGARET TAIT

Introduction

There are now many specially designed assessments which give information on the progress of children with cochlear implants, once they have understanding and use of spoken language. For example, their speech perception skills can be evaluated by testing their recognition of words in closed and open set (Osberger et al., 1991a), and the quality of their speech can be assessed (Miyamoto et al., 1992). The assessment of prelingually deafened children, or those who have completely lost any language they had acquired, requires less direct techniques. Some of these children may have begun to understand and use sign language, and would not, therefore, be prelinguistic; however, all of them would be considered to be pre-verbal, as having no understanding or use of spoken language. This means that we can neither assess their auditory reception of words nor the clarity and extent of their speech. Yet the assessment of these children is as important as that of children who have developed spoken language.

Research in the last 15 years has identified several distinct, sequential stages which normally hearing infants pass through before the emergence of verbal communication. These stages form the foundations of spoken language and include two important features of interaction. One is the ability to distribute attention between the parent and objects of communication (Collis, 1977). Quite early in life – around 4–6 months – the infant begins to follow the parent's line of gaze, just as the parent has been doing for the infant. Such shared visual attention to objects in the environment helps infants to discover the significance of what is being said to them. The other important ingredient of early communication is the development of the ability to take turns in dialogue – the normal practice in conversation. This aspect develops before the child begins to talk (Bruner, 1983) and includes the use of intentional bodily gestures such as pointing (Zinober and Martlew, 1985).

Comparable research into the pre-verbal development of deaf children indicates that the achievement of similar sequential stages predates the emergence of verbal communication (Wood et al., 1986; Tait and Wood, 1987). Deaf children, too, need to develop the ability to distribute their visual attention (we call this 'eye contact', or 'visual regard') and to take turns in dialogue ('turn-taking'). Good acoustic hearing aid amplification is known to promote the development of these early spoken language skills (Ling and Ling, 1978; Clark, 1989). It is necessary to know that the implant and speech processor are fulfilling a similar function for those children who have insufficient hearing to use acoustic hearing aids. Observation of the development of pre-verbal skills will show whether or not they are receiving appropriate auditory information from the speech processor.

Assessment of these skills as they develop is greatly assisted by video analysis. Video recordings of each child in interaction with a known adult, made at regular intervals, will enable the monitoring of development, over time, of eye contact and conversational turn-taking. Auditory awareness and processing skills (the child's reaction to and interpretation of the sound of speech) can also be monitored through video analysis, by observing how a child reacts to speech when not looking at the speaker. In Nottingham a well-documented method of video analysis (Tait, 1987; Tait and Wood, 1987) is used to assess the pre-verbal and early verbal development of the cochlear implantees who are implanted while at a pre-verbal stage. This chapter describes the procedure, discusses ways in which the analysis can provide indications of the effect of the implant on the child's communication, and includes three illustrative cases. The methods are also discussed in Tait (1993).

Setting up the video: lighting, sound quality, frequency and length

Lighting

The room used for making the video needs to be light enough to make a clear recording. If the natural illumination is not sufficient, some form of extra lighting needs to be arranged and this should be placed discretely so that the child is not dazzled. However, making a video in daylight is usually possible. It is best to film away from the window with the child sideways on to it, so that the light falls on his or her face without having to look directly into it. This gives sufficient illumination to see the direction of the child's gaze when making the transcript. The camera needs to be pointing mainly at the child, but also taking in the adult in profile. The child needs to be seen almost full face to be sure of the direction and focus of his gaze, whereas a profile view of the adult is sufficient to be able to tell where she is looking, her facial expression, and any signs, gestures or body language. (To avoid confusion, wherever possible 'she' is used to refer to the adult and 'he' to the child.)

Sound quality

The room in which the video is made should be reasonably quiet. This may seem obvious, but with normal hearing it is easy to overlook background noise which will make listening difficult for the child, and also for the person doing the transcription afterwards. For the same reasons, a reverberant room is not ideal either. Very often the filming can take place in the child's home, where soft furnishings provide a good acoustical environment.

Frequency and length of video sessions

In Nottingham video films are made at the following intervals:

- preimplant (two separate occasions)
- postimplant (within the first 2 weeks after initial tuning)
- 3 months after initial tuning
- 6 months after initial tuning
- 12 months after initial tuning, and thereafter only if necessary.

Filming lasts for between 5 and 10 minutes (longer only if there is difficulty in establishing normal interaction) with the aim of eventually transcribing no more than 5 minutes. This has been found to be long enough to get a good impression of the quality of interaction of which a child is capable, and it is also important to avoid prolonging the labour-intensive and time-consuming business of transcription unnecessarily.

Content of session

This depends on the age and communication ability of the child, but whatever stage he is at, the aim is to monitor what is emerging, not to enforce change. When filming, it is necessary to be guided by the child's role in the interaction, following his line of interest and trying to interpret what is in his mind rather than expecting him to interpret what is in the adult's mind – in other words, to be as normal and child-centred as possible. When dealing with a child who is in the early stages, without much (or any) receptive and expressive language, it is helpful to include a 'format' (Bruner, 1983), i.e. a situation which has within it the possibility of enjoyable predictability. For example, toys such as a jack-in-the-box, toy train plus people, farm trailer plus sheep and cows, are all capable of being used in this way. These predictable shared activities solve, or at least make easier for the child, the problem of where to look and when to take a turn, and make the interaction relaxed and enjoyable. Similar situations can be used both before and after implantation, so that the videos can be compared.

An example of such a situation, using a farm vehicle and animals, is given below. The adult's and the child's 'turns' are presented in sequence (A = adult; C = child).

A: Go, lorry, round, that's right. You'll have to tell it to –
C: [gestures 'stop']
A: – to stop, that's right. Can you –
C: – [points at empty driver's cab]
A: What's in there? No, there's no little man, is there, driving it, no. Stop, lorry. Get out, sheep. Now then, which of those shall we have?
C: [picks up cow]
A: A cow. The cow says   'Moooo, moooo, moooo}
C: Moooo,   mooooo}
A: He wants a ride, Moooo.
C: [gestures 'sleep']
A: Go to sleep, that's right, go to sleep, cow.

Once the animal game has been initiated, the adult in this example is prepared to follow the child's lead at any point. From the way in which the child takes his 'turns' it is clear that he feels an equal partner in the interaction; he interrupts the adult twice, and by gestures ('stop' and 'sleep') suggests what is to happen next. It is also useful, particularly after the initial tuning sessions have taken place, to spend part of the time looking at a book. This is because it will be more natural for the child to look at the book than at the adult, and so the beginnings of auditory processing will become apparent – for example, in his repetition (without looking) of something the adult has just said. It may be more difficult to get that information in a set-up where adult and child are facing each other, if the child has already established the habit of looking at the speaker's face.

Measures

Progress in pre-verbal development is monitored in the following areas

Turn-taking

- Turn-taking involving gesture/sign.
- Turn-taking involving voice and, eventually, words.

Autonomy

- Vocal turn which cannot be predicted from adult's preceding turn (see below).
- Gestural turn which cannot be predicted from the adult's preceding turn.

Eye contact

- Eye contact with the speaker.
- Division of visual attention between speaker and object of reference.

Auditory awareness

Indications of auditory awareness in the following:

- Repetitions (unsolicited) of words when not in eye contact with the adult.
- Vocal turn-taking after not having been in eye contact with the adult.

Making and analysing the transcript

Three transcripts (Figures 10.1, 10.2 and 10.3) show the scoring in detail.

Turn-taking

This is marked on the transcript by an arrow every time it is clear that the adult has left a pause for the child to take part, or when the child has interrupted the adult's turn. It is useful, particularly when first using this approach, for two people to look separately at the video, to see if there is reasonable agreement as to the points at which turns have been left. (The reliability of the Nottingham analysis has already been established by a replicability study: Tait, 1984). The total number of turns is then counted, the number of turns taken by gesture or by vocalisation is counted, and the latter are then expressed as percentages of the total number of turns. Figure 10.1 shows how this works out in practice.

The adult has left three turns – occasions when she has paused, still looking at the child, to give him the chance to take part if he wishes. (Of course, a child may decide to take a turn where he has not been left an opening, in which case the adult should give way to him.) How does the child in Figure 10.1 take the turns he is offered?

- On the first he does not respond.
- On the second he responds with a gesture.

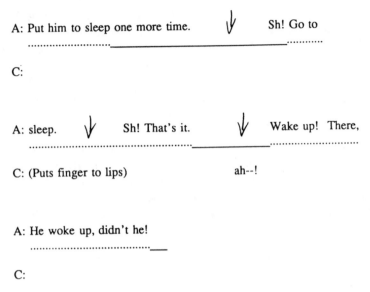

A: Put him to sleep one more time.   ↓   Sh! Go to

C:

A: sleep.   ↓   Sh! That's it.   ↓   Wake up! There,

C: (Puts finger to lips)   ah--!

A: He woke up, didn't he!

C:

Figure 10.1 Transcript of conversational interaction, illustrating turn-taking. Adult's and child's contributions are presented in parallel. Dotted and solid lines indicate eye contact (see text). Arrows mark the pauses left for the child's conversational turns

- On the third he vocalises.

Therefore, his responses have been as follows:

- Gesture on one out of three occasions: 33%
- Voice on one out of three occasions: 33%
- No response on one out of three occasions: 33%

When monitoring a child's progress after implantation, earlier sessions can be compared with later sessions, to see whether, for example, vocal turn-taking is increasing.

Autonomy

We can also look at the amount of autonomy the child is showing in this situation. Is he simply repeating what the adult has said, and giving predictable responses to closed questions, or is he taking his turns in a manner which cannot be predicted from the adult's preceding turn, and showing progress towards more normal interaction? Examples of autonomy could include introducing new topics or information, contradicting the adult, joking, asking questions, and so on. The amount of autonomy he is able to exert will depend largely on the adult's conversational style; if she is very 'controlling', for example, asking a lot of closed questions, the child may not be able to show the autonomy of which he is capable.

The child's use of autonomy can be assessed by counting the number of turns in which he offers something that cannot be directly predicted from the adult's preceding remark, and then expressing that number as a percentage of the total number of turns. In this way we can see how much autonomy is being exercised vocally and how much gesturally. The child in Figure 10.1 does not show any autonomy. He takes part in the interaction which has been initiated by the adult, but does not take control or change its course in any way. His percentage of autonomy is therefore 0%. Another child's use of autonomy is illustrated in Figure 10.2. Here there are four turns, in three of which the child speaks, and in one of which she shakes her head. Therefore:

- She responds vocally on three out of four occasions: 75%
- She responds gesturally on one out of four occasions: 25%

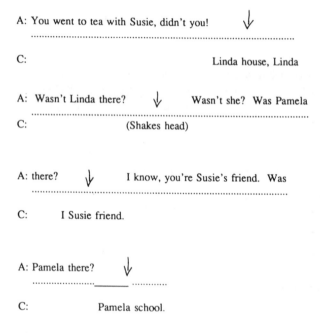

Figure 10.2 Transcript of conversational interaction, illustrating child autonomy (see text). Dotted and solid lines indicate eye contact (see text). Arrows mark the occasions when the child takes a conversational turn

Her exercise of autonomy in the three vocal turns is as follows:

- In the first she introduces new information.
- In the second she insists on correcting what she sees as lack of understanding on the adult's part – she has gone to tea with Susie, not her sister.

- In the third she goes beyond the adult's closed question to give additional information.

Therefore on each of these occasions she shows autonomy: 75%, expressed as a percentage of the total number of turns. Her gestural turn does not show autonomy, being a simple nod of the head. This child is exercising autonomy through the use of actual words, but autonomy can be observed in a child's vocal turns before he has reached the stage of being able to use words. He may, for example, vocalise forcefully to draw the adult's attention to something.

Visual regard

The child's visual regard – the direction of his gaze and focus of his attention – needs to be shown on the transcript. This is a time-consuming activity, but very revealing. Instances which are very fleeting on the video film can be documented, affording more lengthy and detailed scrutiny.

The visual regard is added to the transcript as a dotted line just under the adult's words (or parts of words) for which the child *is* looking at her, and as a continuous line at a lower level under the words for which he is *not* looking (i.e. when he is looking at the object of discourse or elsewhere). At the latter points the focus of his attention is noted, in brackets. The total number of the adult's syllables is counted, then the number of syllables for which the child is looking at the adult. The latter ('looking' syllables) is expressed as a percentage of the former (total number of syllables).

This gives a broad measure, but the child's gaze can be examined in greater detail. For example, is he getting to be more likely to look away at the end of the adult's speaking turn instead of randomly during her turn? Are his glances towards the object of interest becoming more fleeting and his looks towards the adult more sustained?

Answers to these questions are illustrated in Figure 10.1:

- A count of the adult's syllables gives a total of 23. The child is looking at her for 19 of these. Therefore his percentage of visual regard of the adult in this tiny excerpt is 83%.
- The focus of his attention is relevant. Each time he looks away from the adult he looks at the puppet, so that he is always looking at either the speaker or the object of interest.
- In this familiar situation he is becoming more likely to look away from the adult at the end of her speaking turn, rather than in the middle of it, and to return quickly after he has looked away. His looking at the adult is therefore well sustained.

Auditory processing

One of the clearest indications of auditory processing is that the child begins to take vocal turns when he has broken eye contact with the adult during her preceding turns, i.e. he has looked away from her while she was speaking, and yet still comes in with a vocalisation when she pauses to leave him a conversational turn. This suggests that he is beginning to register auditorily the points at which the adult stops speaking. Each turn is therefore classified according to whether the child has, or has not, been in eye contact just before it – i.e. for the teacher's last few words. Then the percentage of 'non-looking' turns that have been filled vocally by the child is noted, and also the percentage of 'looking' turns that have been filled. If the child is not using auditory processing he is much more likely to fill the 'looking' than the 'non-looking' turns. As auditory processing develops he becomes progressively more likely to fill either sort of turn (Tait, 1984). Looking and non-looking turns are illustrated in Figure 10.3. In the transcript shown in Figure 10.3 there are five turns taken vocally:

- The first is a non-looking turn. Although the child is looking at the adult when he actually says 'car', he has not been looking at her for her previous words.

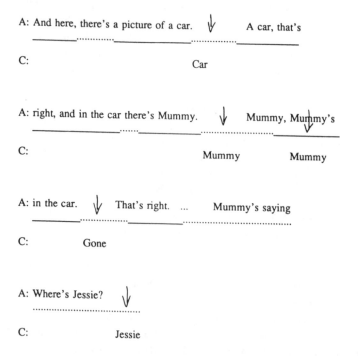

Figure 10.3 Transcript of conversational interaction, illustrating auditory processing, shown by the taking of non-looking turns (see text)

- The second is also a non-looking turn, in the same way.
- The third is a looking turn, occurring simultaneously with the adult's.
- The fourth is another non-looking turn.
- The fifth is a looking turn, because he has been looking at the adult for the latter half of her preceding turn.

Therefore his percentage of non-looking turns during this excerpt is 60%, and of looking turns 40%.

This child is beginning to use attempts at words, but the taking of non-looking vocal turns can be observed before actual words begin to emerge. Another noticeable indication of auditory processing is any repetition (unasked) of something the adult has said when the child was not looking at her. There are two examples of this in Figure 10.3 – the child attempts repetitions of 'car' and 'Mummy', not having been in eye contact with the adult for either of these.

An early indication of the child's awareness of the sound of the adult's voice may be observed in his glancing up when the adult starts to speak, raises her voice or uses an exaggerated intonation pattern, without any visual cue being given. An additional indication may be the development of intonation. In young deaf children who are acoustic hearing aid users, modulation of pitch in their voices is significantly related both to their hearing acuity and to their ability to identify words by listening alone (Tait, 1984). It is possible that in cochlear implantees, too, the development of varied voice pitch may indicate efficient processing of sound.

Illustrative cases

The progress of three children, who by the time of implantation had very different communication skills, is outlined here to illustrate the method. The first, 'Brenda', already had good eye contact and some silent communication in signs. She might be described as being pre-verbal, but not 'pre-language'. The second, 'Martin', had very poor pre-verbal skills and little use of gesture. The third, 'Fiona', was congenitally deaf, with fairly good eye contact and some silent communication by gesture.

Brenda

Brenda was deafened at 1;2 years, and thereafter total communication was used with her by her parents and teacher (i.e. spoken language supported by signing was used by the adults in contact with Brenda and she wore powerful hearing aids, which gave her awareness of sound at a vibrotactile level only). Brenda's understanding and use of signs was well established by the time of the implant operation, when she was aged 2;8 years. She used signs in one- or two-element combinations with considerable autonomy, and rarely vocalised. Figure 10.4 displays her vocal and gestural turn-taking and autonomy, over time. Her use of vocalisation (which 6 months after initial tuning consisted entirely of actual words) increased over time. Vocal autonomy started off more slowly but also increased materially over time. Conversely, turns taken by signing alone (i.e. without vocalisation) decreased over the same period. By the second pre-implant session her visual regard was well established and structured, in that she was more likely to look away at the end of the adult's speaking turn than randomly during the turn. By the 12-month session (i.e. 12 months after initial tuning), when conversing with her mother without any visual aids to meaning, she maintained steady eye contact with her mother, and there were therefore few opportunities to observe auditory processing in non-looking turns. However, in the postimplant, 3-month and 6-month sessions, this information was available, the percentages of non-looking turns for those sessions being 63%, 33% and 62% respectively.

The two transcripts shown in Figures 10.5 and 10.6 demonstrate the changes in her communication. The first (Figure 10.5) is from the second preimplant session. Brenda communicates by silent signing, shown in brackets, and the adult communicates in speech, signing the key words (signing not shown).

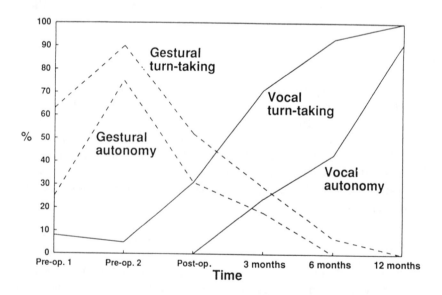

Figure 10.4 Measures of first illustrative case: Brenda. Variations in percentages of vocal and signed turn-taking and autonomy over the period from before implantation to 12 months after implantation

A: That's all right.   ↓   Oh, right! There's no -
_____........._____...

C: (Signs: go away, handle)

A: no handle.   ↓   Yes, it's rubbish, isn't it, go away bucket!
....____

C: (S. go away, rubbish)

A ↓   Go away, you're no good.   ↓   Those are both all
____.................._____...............

C: (Nods)   (S. all right)

A: right, aren't they, they're both the same.   ↓   That's
........._____..................

C: (S. go away)

A: rubbish, yes, that's rubbish.
....

C:

Figure 10.5 Transcript of excerpt from Brenda's second preimplant session

This extract from a longer transcript (5 minutes) demonstrates Brenda's ability to communicate in signs, her willingness to take the lead in the interaction, and her facility in dividing her gaze between speaker and object of discourse. The percentages were as follows:

Sign/gesture turn-taking: 100% (percentage for complete session: 90%)
Sign/gesture autonomy: 80% (percentage for complete session: 75%)
Visual regard: 70% (percentage for complete session: 65%)

The second excerpt, shown in Figure 10.6, is from the session 12 months after initial tuning. The adult is now communicating solely in speech. Brenda signs most of the words she says (signing not shown).

A: What about Joan and Kathy?   ↓

C: Joan, Kathy. Long -- way--

A: It would be a long way, yes.   ↓   Oh, too hard to walk.

C: Hard walk.

A: How would we get there?   ↓   Long way to

C: Long way Kathy House.

A: Kathy's - oh, it's even further than that.   ↓   Very

C: Hard (Signs: walk)

A: hard to walk, yes. How would we get on holidays?   ↓

C: Better in

A: Better to go in the car, that's right, yes, I think so too.

C: car.

Figure 10.6 Transcript excerpt from Brenda's 12-month session. Arrows mark child's conversational turns, which are all taken by words, plus signing (not shown). Adult does not use sign

What is most noticeable here is the complete change-over, in turn-taking and autonomy, from silent signing to speech, with or without the addition of signs. There was no great change in visual regard, which was already well established, except that by this 12-month stage she displayed the pattern of eye contact normal to adult conversation –

i.e. she looked at the person who was talking to her, and looked away when she was speaking herself. There was one indication of auditory processing – she was not looking at her mother when the latter said 'Joan', but repeated it. Percentages for turn-taking, autonomy and visual regard were as follows:

Vocal turn-taking:	100% (percentage for complete session: 100%)
Vocal autonomy:	100% (percentage for complete session: 91%)
Visual regard:	85% (percentage for complete session: 85%)

During this 12-month period Brenda had received systematic tuning of the device and monthly habilitation sessions (fortnightly in the period immediately after the initial tuning sessions) where listening activities were pursued, leading to awareness and discrimination of speech features, together with interactions fostering the development of vocal communication. There was at all times close liaison between the staff responsible for the tuning of the device and the cochlear implant rehabilitation staff who also worked closely with the parents and local professionals.

Martin

Martin was deafened at 2;8 years, and an oral approach was used by his parents and teachers, well supplemented by natural gestures and facial expression. He had lost all his understanding and use of spoken language, and seemed to have equal difficulty making sense of gesture. His visual regard and turn-taking were at a very low level and there were only very moderate increases over a preoperative period of 6 months. He was implanted at the age of 3;5 years.

Figure 10.7 displays his vocal and gestural turn-taking and autonomy, over time. It shows his development of pre-verbal and early verbal skills over the 12-month period after initial tuning. His visual regard increased over the first 6 months, as pre-verbal skills became established, and then decreased as Martin gradually began to rely less on visual contact where his own turn-taking was concerned. This was also shown by a rise over time in non-looking turns, the percentages for the post-initial stimulation, 3-month, 6-month and 12-month sessions being 33%, 56%, 50% and 73% respectively. Vocal turn-taking increased steadily over the whole period, whereas turn-taking by gesture tailed off.

Two transcripts demonstrate the changes in his pre-verbal skills and early verbal communication. Both complete transcripts were 5 minutes in length. The first excerpt is from the second preimplant session, and is shown in Figure 10.8.

Martin was engaged in the interaction to the extent that he was looking at the object of discourse, but his visual regard of the adult was

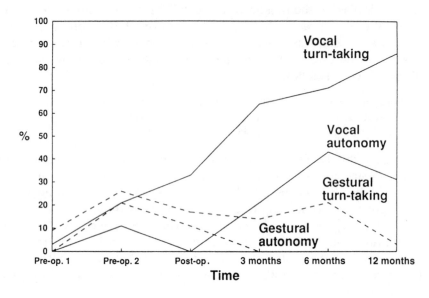

Figure 10.7 Measures of second illustrative case: Martin. The variation in percentages of vocal and gestural turn-taking and autonomy over the period from before implantation to 12 months after implantation

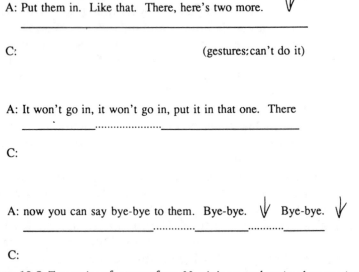

Figure 10.8 Transcript of excerpt from Martin's second preimplant session

at a low level. His turn-taking was also at a low level, and entirely by gesture except on the two occasions (not shown) when reluctant voice was coaxed from him by offering the microphone. What autonomy there was also came via gesture. Percentages for turn-taking, autonomy and visual regard were as follows:

Gesture turn-taking: 33% (percentage for complete session: 26%)
Gesture autonomy: 33% (percentage for complete session: 21%)
Visual regard: 17% (percentage for complete session: 18%)

The second excerpt is from the session 12 months after initial tuning, and is shown in Figure 10.9. Having acquired the pre-verbal visual regard skills, Martin showed at the 12-month stage that he was able to come in with his own vocal turn whether or not he had been looking at the adult for her turn, and to be capable of adding something new to the conversation. Percentages for turn-taking, autonomy, visual regard and non-looking turns were as follows:

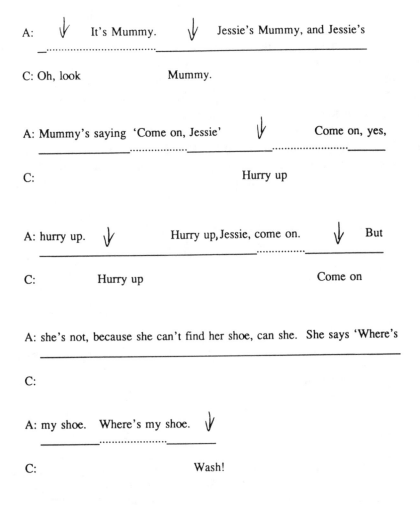

Figure 10.9 Transcript of excerpt from Martin's 12-month session. Arrows mark child's conversational turns, all of which are taken by words, without gesture

Vocal turn-taking:	100% (percentage for complete session: 86%)
Vocal autonomy:	50% (percentage for complete session: 31%)
Visual regard:	20% (percentage for complete session: 34%)
Non-looking turns:	67% (percentage for complete session: 73%)

As was the case with Brenda (and with all the children implanted at Nottingham), Martin had received regular tuning of the device during this 12-month period. He had already been monitored by video analysis for 6 months before implantation, during which period development of pre-verbal skills was extremely slow. His progress after initial tuning was material, with steady increase in the pre-verbal skills which were necessary for his development of speech.

Fiona

Fiona was born profoundly deaf. Diagnosis and provision of hearing aids took place when she was 5 months old, but she derived little benefit from amplified sound, her awareness being only at a vibrotactile level. At the time of the implant operation she was aged 4;5 years. An oral approach had been used by parents and teachers, but Fiona communicated mainly by silent gestures plus occasional vocalisations. Figure 10.10 displays her vocal and gestural turn-taking and autonomy, over time, and shows how Fiona's use of vocalisation, which by 6 months consisted almost entirely of actual words, increased over time.

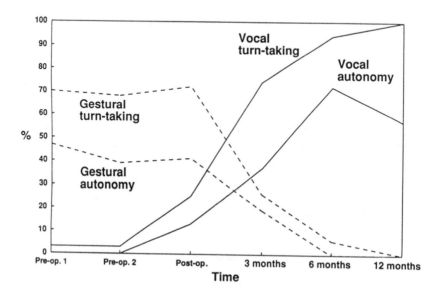

Figure 10.10 Measures of third illustrative case: Fiona. Variations in percentages of vocal and signed turn-taking and autonomy over the period from before implantation to 12 months after implantation

Her use of vocal autonomy shows a comparable increase. Conversely, gestural turn-taking and autonomy decrease over time. Her eye contact, 18% at the first preimplant session, increases steadily over time, to 63% at 12 months. Non-looking turns go from 0% preimplant to 50% postimplant, and remain around that level. The two transcripts shown in Figures 10.11 and 10.12 demonstrate the changes in her communication. The first, from the second preimplant session, shows Fiona communicating by silent gesture. This excerpt from a longer session demonstrates Fiona's willingness to communicate by gesture and her readiness to take the lead in the interaction. The percentages were as follows:

Gestural turn-taking: 80% (percentage for complete session: 68%)
Gestural autonomy: 60% (percentage for complete session: 39%)
Visual regard: 27% (percentage for complete session: 31%)

The second excerpt, shown in Figure 10.12, is from the session 12 months after initial tuning. As with Brenda, what is most noticeable is the complete change-over from silent gesture to speech, both in turn-taking and use of autonomy. Four of her five turns are non-looking, showing the development of auditory processing. Her percentages for vocal turn-taking, vocal autonomy and visual regard are as follows:

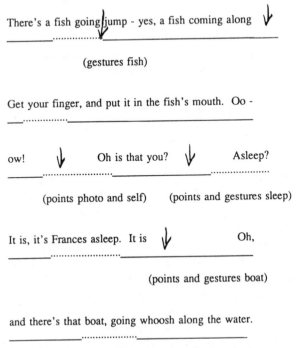

There's a fish going jump - yes, a fish coming along

(gestures fish)

Get your finger, and put it in the fish's mouth. Oo -

ow!   Oh is that you?   Asleep?

(points photo and self)   (points and gestures sleep)

It is, it's Frances asleep. It is   Oh,

(points and gestures boat)

and there's that boat, going whoosh along the water.

Figure 10.11 Transcript of excerpt from Fiona's second preimplant session. Arrows mark the child's conversational turns, which are all taken by silent gesture, shown in brackets

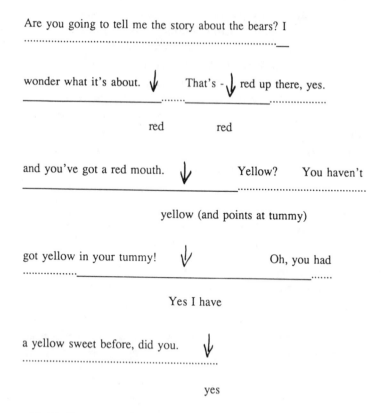

Are you going to tell me the story about the bears? I

wonder what it's about. ↓   That's - ↓ red up there, yes.

red   red

and you've got a red mouth. ↓   Yellow?   You haven't

yellow (and points at tummy)

got yellow in your tummy! ↓   Oh, you had

Yes I have

a yellow sweet before, did you. ↓

yes

Figure 10.12 Transcript of excerpt from Fiona's 12-month session. Arrows mark the child's conversational turns, which are all taken by words

Vocal turn-taking: 100% (percentage for complete session: 100%)
Vocal autonomy: 80% (percentage for complete session: 57%)
Visual regard: 62% (percentage for complete session: 63%)

Fiona was the first of the congenitally deaf children to be implanted at Nottingham. At 4;5 years she was one of the older of the pre-verbal children, and, of course, had never had effective auditory stimulation. It is interesting that her progress is comparable with that of Brenda, who heard until she was 1;2 years, and who was implanted at 2;8 years. The experience of this child and that of the other congenitally deaf children in the Nottingham programme lead to the belief that, over time, the benefit for them may be as great as for those who have had some experience of sound. This belief is substantiated by the findings of Osberger and colleagues (1991c) who reported that there was no obvious difference in speech perception abilities between children with implants who were born deaf and those who had hearing for 1–3 years before onset of deafness.

Assessing children's progress

Turn-taking

As children's transcripts are looked at over time, it is hoped at Nottingham that development of vocal turn-taking and autonomy will be seen, and that use of silent sign and gesture will fall away. These developments have been noticeable with the pre-verbal children in Nottingham's Paedriatric Cochlear Implant Programme. Figure 10.13 shows the development of vocal turn-taking over the 12 months following initial tuning of the processor for all the pre-verbal children who have reached that stage in the programme. These numbered 16, including 3 who were congenitally deaf. Before implantation, nine of these children were to some extent using silent sign and gesture to communicate. Seven, on the other hand, were as poor communicators in sign or gesture as they were in speech. It is interesting that silent turn-taking fell away equally noticeably in the case of those children who before implantation were using it in a high percentage of their turns, as in the case of those who were not communicating in this way. Some did continue to use signs, but always accompanied first by voice and later by words.

It is not only the frequency of vocalisation that is being looked for as evidence that children are becoming vocal, but also indications that the vocalisations are becoming increasingly varied and word-like. The

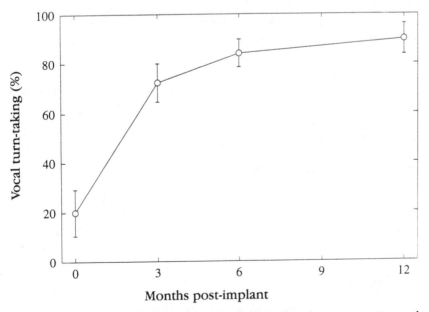

Figure 10.13 Variations in the percentage of vocal turn-taking (see text) over the period from before implantation to 12 months after implantation, for 16 children

Analysis of Spontaneous Speech Samples (Osberger et al., 1991b) has been used by the Nottingham team's speech and language therapist on the same transcripts, and has helped to identify a child with a specific language problem.

Visual regard

Development of eye contact is very idiosyncratic, but by looking at the transcripts over time it is hoped that the findings will show that children are progressively finding appropriate levels of visual regard in various communicative situations, i.e. they show increased facility in distributing their attention, are able to sustain eye contact when necessary, and are able to react to what is being said while looking at the object of discourse. The visual regard percentage needs to be related to that of vocal turn-taking when assessing children's progress. Low eye contact is not necessarily a counter-indication of linguistic progress if at the same time the child's vocal turns display increasing frequency, variety and autonomy, and word-like vocalisations are emerging. However, if this is not the case, low eye contact may be a cause for concern, particularly if the ability to sustain eye contact and to refer from speaker to object of discourse does not appear to be developing.

Auditory processing

Looking at transcripts over time one would expect to see children taking a greater proportion of non-looking turns, thus displaying less dependence on the visual channel for communication. All the pre-verbal children at Nottingham showed a material increase in their percentage of non-looking turns within the first few months after the initial tuning sessions. However, this measure needs to be related to vocal turn-taking, because it is not meaningful unless there is a reasonable number of vocal turns. If, for example, a child only took two or three turns vocally, his looking or not looking just before these points could be a matter of chance.

Present research

Examination of the pattern of the measures obtained from video analysis (vocal and gestural turn-taking and autonomy, eye contact and non-looking turns) in children with cochlear implants and children with acoustic hearing aids is under way.

Conclusions

Progress towards understanding and use of spoken language, through audition, cannot be predicted before implantation, and it is vital to monitor indications of development as they occur. It is, therefore, important to transcribe the videos within a short time of making the recordings and to video all pre-verbal children. The measures used – vocal turn-taking, vocal autonomy and non-looking turns in particular – are sensitive indicators of use of the implant system. It has been found at Nottingham that percentages in these measures have fallen sharply if for any reason there has not been consistent use of the processor.

Even with consistent use, progress measured in understanding and use of actual words can be very slow where young pre-verbal children are concerned. The techniques of video analysis make it possible to observe minute changes over time in turn-taking and auditory processing. The analysis provides objective evidence, before children are able to undertake formal speech and language evaluations, that there is, or is not, progress in the preverbal skills which are the pre-requisite of spoken language.

References

Bruner, J.S. (1983). *Child's Talk: Learning to Use Language*. Oxford: Oxford University Press.

Clark, M. (1989). *Language Through Living*. London: Hodder & Stoughton.

Collis, G.M. (1977). Visual co-orientation in maternal speech. In H.R. Schaffer (ed.), *Studies in Mother-Infant Interaction*. London: Academic Press.

Ling, D. and Ling, A. (1978). *Aural Habilitation*. Washington DC: Alexander Graham Bell Association for the Deaf.

Miyamoto, R.T., Osberger, M.J., Robbins, M.S., Myers, W.A., Kessler, K. and Pope, M.L. (1992). Longitudinal evaluation of communication skills of children with single- or multi-channel cochlear implants. *American Journal of Otology*, **13**, 215–222.

Osberger, M.J., Miyamoto, R.T., Zimmerman-Phillips, M.S., Kemink, J.L., Stroer, B.S., Firszt, J.B. and Novak, M.A. (1991a). Independent evaluation of the speech perception abilities of children with the Nucleus 22-channel cochlear implant system. *Ear and Hearing*, **12**, (Suppl. 4), 66–80.

Osberger, M.J., Robbins, M.S., Berry, S.W., Todd, S.L., Hesketh, M.S. and Allison Sedey, M.A. (1991b). Analysis of the spontaneous speech samples of children with cochlear implants or tactile aids. *American Journal of Otology*, **12** (Suppl.), 151–164.

Osberger, M.J., Todd, S.L., Berry, S.W., Robbins, A.M. and Miyamoto, R.T. (1991c). Effect of age at onset of deafness on children's speech perception abilities with a cochlear implant. *Annals of Otology, Rhinology and Laryngology*, **100**, 883–888.

Tait, D.M. (1984). The role of singing in the social and linguistic development of nursery-aged deaf children. Unpublished PhD thesis, University of Nottingham.

Tait, D.M. (1987). Making and monitoring progress in the pre-school years. *Journal of British Association of Teachers of the Deaf*, **11**(5), 143–153.

Tait, D.M. (1993). Video analysis: A method of assessing changes in pre-verbal and early linguistic communication following cochlear implantation. *Ear and Hearing*, **14** (6), 378–389.

Tait, D.M. and Wood, D.J. (1987). From communication to speech in deaf children.

Child Language Teaching and Therapy, **3** (1), 1–16.

Wood, D.J., Wood, H., Griffiths, A.J. and Howarth, I. (1986). *Teaching and Talking with Deaf Children.* Chichester: John Wiley & Sons.

Zinober, B. and Martlew, M. (1985). The Development of communicative gestures. In M.D. Barrett (ed.), *Children's Single Word Speech*, pp. 183–215. Chichester: John Wiley & Sons.

Chapter 11
Monitoring progress: the role of a speech and language therapist

DEE DYAR

This chapter will consider the following aspects involved in monitoring progress: the principles of effective casework as influenced by practice in established paediatric programmes and the views of parents of deaf children; measurement issues and the establishment of baseline criteria; the classification of linguistic status of deaf children before and after implantation; a suggested speech and language assessment battery for young profoundly deaf children; factors which influence the rate of progress after implantation with some examples of practice; and finally, identified gaps in current practice and future trends in service delivery.

The considerations are based on the literature, recent conference proceedings on paediatric implantation issues and trends and the insights gained in actual practice as a member of the Nottingham Paediatric Cochlear Implant Programme. The philosophy of this implant team is to provide a seamless management regime. This implies a flexible and stress-free programme of care for the child, family and local professionals. In the case of young implanted deaf children the purposes of monitoring progress by the implant team speech and language therapist (SLT) are the following:

- To *assess* and *describe* the individual child's current communication skills and ongoing needs before implantation.
- To *document* an individual child's progress in communication skills over time after implantation and to provide progress updates on all children within the implant programme at agreed assessment intervals.
- To *investigate* the possibility of unforeseen non-sensory difficulties in the case of deaf children who present as 'under-functioning' as users of a single or multichannel implant.
- To *observe* the child in a range of everyday settings as well as in performance-based tasks, to guarantee the representative nature of assessment findings.

- To *share* information and appropriate advice on strategies to develop the child's communication skills with his or her family and a range of local professionals, and by doing so to complement the work of the implant team teachers of the deaf in particular.
- To *contribute* to team evaluation and monitoring procedures by providing information to the team coordinator on SLT assessment and intervention outcomes, data analysis and aspects of outreach programmes.

In addition to the identified priorities, a team SLT may be requested to contribute to team-initiated research and investigations on targeted groups of implanted children, for example, pre-verbal or low-verbal deaf children. This may involve the need to substantiate the use of a 'descriptive' approach as a precursor to norm-referenced or criterion-referenced performance measures. Along with the audiological scientist and teacher of the deaf, a team SLT may be called upon to identify factors which may have a high correlation to successful use of the device. Again, an SLT may implement innovative research-based sampling measures, such as video analysis, into everyday team practice. It is important that objective measurements of speech and voice skills are obtained even in the case of young deaf children. This may mean that computer-based programs resource materials and presentation formats need to be adapted by an SLT in collaboration with other professionals.

A team-based SLT will share a commitment to more uniform data collection across different languages and cultures, by paediatric implant programmes to promote the exchange of information at an international level (Table 11.1).

Table 11.1 Role of a team speech–language therapist

Pre-selection	Advisory
	Indirect contact with child/family
Selection	Comprehensive assessment of the child's communication skills
Switch-on	Establish casework relationship with family and local professionals at implant centre and in local setting
	Written report
0–1 year interval	Direct contact with child at implant centre and at home/school
	Ongoing assessment at 3 months, 6 months and 12 months
	Indirect contact with family and local professionals – live, telephone or written, as required
	Written progress report
1–3 year interval	As above
4 year interval	Annual review at implant centre
	Written report
5 year interval	Annual review at implant centre
	Written progress

Ways of working

The development of a paediatric cochlear implant programme has already been described (Chapter 3). The recommended frequency, content and nature of an effective outreach programme must also be described so that the long-term needs of the deaf child can be met satisfactorily at the local level. This involves the team teacher of the deaf and the SLT in sharing skills and exchanging information, advice, reassurance and support with a range of local professionals. The purposes of monitoring the progress of a deaf child after cochlear implantation will vary according to the professional background of the team scientist, educator or SLT. For this reason it is important that a paediatric cochlear implant programme adopts a genuinely 'interdisciplinary' rather than multidisciplinary management approach. An interdisciplinary management approach implies a child-centred way of working, and planned opportunities to share insights and concerns with team colleagues as well as with the child's family and the professionals involved. On the other hand, a multidisciplinary approach may simply mean a number of professionals working in parallel. This frequently results from split-site locations of work and may appear to be an effective way of working within a discipline, but it can be stressful for the deaf child's family for two reasons. First, the parent has to act as a go-between, sharing assessment outcomes with a number of team-based professionals and, second, the parent may choose to use team-initiated advice selectively in the absence of team collaboration. For these reasons it seems important to stress the rewards of peer support and perspective which result from regular implant team meetings and established feedback systems. Deafness affects everyone in the family. The professional must always keep in mind the notion of a family as a system in which all parts are intimately and inextricably linked (Luterman, 1987). It is important that the team SLT establishes a confident rapport and also an 'active' working relationship with the deaf child's family and local professionals from the start. Implant team professionals must guard against situations that force one to work or to be perceived as an 'expert' rather than a 'specialist resource person'. Traditional practice means that deaf children usually receive speech and language therapy in a clinic or school setting. An emphasis tends to be placed on high levels of direct contact with the child and on an SLT-initiated programme of intervention. In such an example, feedback among professionals, joint planning and rehabilitation sessions may be dependent on the clinic appointment schedule, school timetable, and the goodwill or flexibility of the professionals involved with the child.

An outreach or distance learning programme may be considered a non-traditional way of working. To be effective it requires comprehensive planning and case record keeping by the outreach professional.

Direct contact sessions may be at 2–3 month intervals rather than on a traditional weekly or monthly basis. The SLT, however, may choose to work with the child at school, home or in another setting as appropriate. Siblings and extended family can observe or be involved in rehabilitation programmes. A team SLT will develop and build upon a personal style of working in an outreach programme. Ideally, they should perceive parents and local professionals as partners and co-workers, so that requisite assessments can be made and communication skills objectives can be planned and implemented jointly. To paraphrase Luterman (1987), an outreach professional must be empathetic to the time lag involved before families adjust to the new reality of a deaf child with a cochlear implant. The outreach professional needs to acknowledge the range and diversity of coping strategies used by different families. The following comments are taken from a recorded interview with the mother of a profoundly deaf child in a discussion about speech and language therapy provision.

Speech and language therapy: a parent's view

Live discussion at the time problems and difficulties arise is by far the best.

Joint sessions because they give me a great deal of hope because you can see the improvement. You've always stressed the things he *can* do rather than the things he can't ... It's nice to see them at a time when you say 'Right, that is not happening yet but we can do this and this to make it happen'. So it almost doesn't matter that I'm seeing things he can't do because at the same time I am getting ideas and hope that they will happen.

I like to have the *written reports* but given that I have the other two opportunities, I could do without them.

Once a deaf child has been selected for a cochlear implant the team SLT may receive a live, telephone or written enquiry for help from the child's local SLT. Not all deaf children in the UK are seen for regular speech and language therapy at the local level. Approximately 70% of the implanted children in the Nottingham programme have access to local speech and language therapy. The team-based SLT, however, will become involved with all children in the programme and will provide support and guidance to the deaf child's family and local professionals, as appropriate, in conjunction with the team teacher of the deaf.

An initial enquiry tends to include a number of the following queries and concerns: How much training should a child have before he receives a cochlear implant? What is the role of a team SLT? What is the philosophy of the implant programme in relation to sign-dominant deaf children? Information is also sought on the purpose and nature of an outreach visit by a team SLT, the frequency of such visits, and whether the team SLT prescribes the frequency of contact and the practice of a local SLT. Such questions reflect the commitment as well as the anxiety of a local professional in this relatively new field. Ideally, the team coordinator will have identified and responded to the need to provide appropriate and user-friendly written resource materials and a recommended reading list. The assigned team teacher of the deaf will have made preliminary contact with the family and local professionals, and usually will have started an awareness training programme in the local setting before a team SLT becomes involved.

The purposes of a SLT working at the outreach or local level may be summarised as follows:

- To document progress and identify the child's ongoing needs in everyday settings.
- To ensure that realistic aims and objectives are being set for recently implanted deaf children.
- To promote collaborative approaches in assessment and monitoring progress during the first few years after implantation.
- To consolidate local understanding and attitudes to the potential benefit of a cochlear implant in an educational setting and in everyday communication.
- To provide reassurance and share skills to implement an appropriate programme of intervention at the local level.

An outreach visit may include a request for an informal presentation by the team SLT. The aims of the team professional when meeting such a request are first to de-mystify the mythology of cochlear implants and deaf children as described by Laurenzi (1993) and second to promote robust everyday classroom management of the implanted child. Experience suggests that, with direction, classmates, like siblings, can be wonderful allies in effecting changes in everyday communication at a realistic and intuitive pace.

At all times the outreach professional encourages contributions from the local teacher of the deaf and support services, for example, written progress reports (see Chapter 9). Establishing an effective local management regime may include altering expectations which may be too high as a result of understandable enthusiasm in the early months after implantation. More surprisingly, it has also been found to be important to raise expectations in the case of some school-aged deaf children when local professionals seem cautious and over-reliant on their knowledge of the child's auditory capabilities before implantation.

As a member of an implant programme, an SLT has the opportunity to work with implanted deaf children of differing ability. Nevertheless it is important to view the recently implanted child through the eyes of the local professionals: they may have been supporting the child's family from the time a diagnosis of deafness was made. De-skilling of local professionals can occur unwittingly, if the team professional projects an image of unattainable expertise when working with the child at the implant centre or on an outreach visit.

Once a working relationship has been established, it is important that the outreach professional negotiates change by demonstrating what the child can do, for example, when speechreading without sign support in closed set tasks, and at a later stage using an implant without lipreading.

An *active* local management regime results from the sharing by the implant team professionals of their implant team assessments, objectives and outcomes in an *accessible* way. For example:

- Using the parent or teachers as the interactor in video samples.
- Sharing video extracts of implanted children at the same stage or at 'attainable' stages of linguistic development.
- Providing a broad outline of aims and goals for the child within a realistic time scale, for example, one school term.
- Arranging planned discussion time to share feelings and to talk through difficult or amorphous sessions as well as sharing more concrete information on ideas, materials and strategies.

Providing an informal written summary of the SLT session outcomes and recommendations on the day of the outreach visit may be helpful. Such guidelines are usually accepted by local professionals when it is pointed out that the aims and objectives are appropriate, realistic and time-effective, and that the teacher or therapist may wish to try out the activities with non-implanted children. The following outline of SLT activities is taken from a computer-based evaluation program known as IMPEVAL (UK). It has been designed specifically for paediatric implant programmes.

Recommendations for minimum programme support for children below 10 years of age were agreed by the local team and put forward for discussion by other paediatric implant programmes in the UK in 1992 (Table 11.2). A review of progress is also made by members of the implant team at year 4 and 5 (Table 11.3).

The amount and nature of support required by the deaf child's family and local professionals may vary in several ways from the support offered to an adult who has *chosen* to have a cochlear implant. Evaluation of local practice over several years suggest a 60:40 weighting of direct and indirect contact in year 1. By year 3 this weighting has been reversed to 40:60 direct and indirect contact to ensure a confident and active local management regime with a gradual reduction in reliance on the visiting team professional thereafter.

Measurement issues

The following factors have been identified as most likely to influence the implant team professional with a responsibility for assessing the young deaf child's communication skills:

Table 11.2 Recommended aspects of provision by a team SLT

IMPEVAL code	Aspect of provision
1	Fitting, adjusting and maintaining hardware No involvement
2	Rehabilitation with child Used by team teachers of the deaf and SLTs. Direct contact with child other than specified under codes 3, 4 and 5
3	Family counselling and education Used by team teachers of the deaf and SLTs – as appropriate
4	Liaison with other agencies Direct contact by an SLT with the child's local teacher of the deaf, mainstream school staff, educational psychologist, non-teaching support staff – as appropriate
5	Assessment and progress Direct contact with the child for assessment purposes Indirect contact with the child, for example, video analysis procedures Completing interviews, rating scales and checklists Documenting outcomes of skilled observation sessions in the classroom Analysis and interpretation of formal assessment Record keeping including data entries Session planning and outcome summaries Progress report writing st specified intervals
6	Audiological assessment Feedback to team professionals as appropriate
7	Medical check No involvement

Table 11.3 Recommendations for minimum implant programme support

	Year 1	Year 2	Year 3
Team TOD			
Implant centre	8 × 3 hours	3 × 3 hours	3 × 3 hours
Home–school	12 × ½ day	6 × 1/2 day	6 × ½ day
Team SLT			
Implant centre	8 × 3 hours	3 × 3 hours	3 × 3 hours
Home–school	6 × ½ day	4 × ½ day	4 × ½ day

TOD, teacher of the deaf; SLT, speech and language therapist.

- *Appropriateness* in relation to the child's age and interest level.
- The *language level* required to complete an assessment procedure with reliability.
- *Time-effectiveness*: its importantce in terms of administration, especially with low-verbal children but also in terms of subsequent analysis and interpretation of data.

- Selected procedures: these should be *repeatable* and afford comparisons over time and with other measures to be made.
- A high level of *inter-user reliability* is recommended. Any adaptations or modifications made to an assessment should be explicit and used consistently by all test users.
- In multidisciplinary work, assessment outcomes at the auditory, cognitive and neurolinguistic levels should be interrelated.

Making an initial judgement of communication skills: the issues

Ruben (1992) points out that measures of language need to take into account the syntax, semantics, prosody and age-appropriateness of the child's language and also reflect the communication style used between his or her primary caregivers. Tyler and Fryauf-Bertschy (1992) outline three general categories for describing the deaf child's communicative style: passive, interested and demanding. They state that many variations of each exist and the same child may exhibit different styles at various times. Wanner and Gleitman (1989) refer to the writings of Bloomfield (1933) and Chomsky (1965) and describe two crucial facts about the human use of language – it is rule governed and creative. Gaps in the current literature on young profoundly deaf children suggest that using outcome measures for the linguistically developed person may be inappropriate in the case of the linguistically developing child.

It is no longer a widely held view that language development is completed between the ages of 18 months and 5 years. It starts much earlier and goes on much longer. In the case of hearing children, for example, speech development is not always completed between 5 and 7 years of age. Language acquisition, however, continues until at least adolescence, (Haynes, 1989). Haynes stresses the need to acknowledge that language develops in different children at different rates and it is linked to non-linguistic advances. She cites five interrelated areas of development: cognitive, perceptual, motor, social and linguistic. Any deficiencies in one or more of these abilities may limit linguistic competence.

Lund and Duchan (1988) outline the following purposes of assessment. The professional needs to establish the following: whether a language problem exists; what is causing the problem?; what are the areas of deficit?; what are the regularities in the child's language performance?; and, finally, what is recommended after assessment for the individual child? Ideally, a comprehensive assessment will include recorded samples of behaviour as well as performance-based measures. Criterion- or norm-referenced procedures may be used with school-aged children. In the case of pre-verbal or low-verbal deaf children, however, the appropriateness of age-equivalent scores, and relative ranking scores, e.g. percentile scores, may be limited and such scores must be interpreted cautiously. The SLT may need to consider *who* needs the test or particular assessment procedure. It is useful to make an informal evaluation of new procedures from the child's perspective in terms of length, complexity and even cultural appropriateness.

Among other reasons for assessment, Dyson (1987) cautions against the use of an assessment as a means of demonstrating the competence of a particular professional, justifying or estimating the merits of a particular developmental test or to reinforce the justifications for professional decisions that have already been made, e.g. a school placement. Dyson also remarks that the traditional view of the need to assess a child's special needs is self-evident: you have to identify needs to be able to meet them. It is important also to emphasise the purpose of rigorous post-intervention measures at both clinical and non-clinical levels.

Implant team professionals should consider whether similar findings reflect the limitations or strengths of assessment test measures or the actual outcome in benefit to the implanted child (Haggard, 1992). Haggard recommends that implant teams need to look at outcomes in terms of language, cognition and communication as a whole. By implication, in the case of young deaf children 'soft' outcomes may be as important as 'hard' outcomes which result from formal procedures, in the early stages of rehabilitation after implantation.

To conclude, assessments must only test what is assessable. A good assessment should allow a range of responses: children of different abilities may give answers of different complexity. An assessment battery should reflect the continuum of abilities ascribed to profoundly deaf children. Before implantation a deaf child may function as partially hearing and at or near age-level peers in linguistic abilities, especially in the case of acquired deafness. Many profoundly deaf children, however, use some form of sign language as a primary means of everyday communication. It is recommended that deaf children should be enabled to respond using a variety of language forms when it is appropriate to do so.

Classification of linguistic status

The literature remains divided on the most appropriate classification categories to use when describing the relationship between the type, nature and the impact of hearing loss. The international classification remains: congenital; prelingual (before chronological age 2 years); perilingual; and postlingual.

Considerable concern continues to exist regarding this classification among implant team members with a responsibility for (re)habilitation.

Likewise the familiar terms 'oral–aural' and 'total communication' used to describe a deaf child's everyday mode of communication may disguise a continuum of effectiveness, which ranges from ideal for the child's current communication status and needs, to well meaning, but inappropriate. This may be for a variety of reasons, not least the impact of the child's profound deafness on us, as interactors (Wood et al., 1986).

The experience of working predominantly with very young, profoundly deaf children during the last few years suggested the need for a more broad classification or framework for interrelated linguistic skills. This should reflect the differing skills of 'prelingual' and bilingual deaf children. It should also cater for the mismatch of linguistic competences which may result from profound deafness of sudden onset in middle or late childhood. These considerations do not seem to be catered for adequately in the traditional classification.

To illustrate this point, informal evaluation of the spoken language skills of the deaf children in the local programme suggested no less than six subgroups at the time of implantation.

Profoundly deaf children may present with a *full phonological repertoire* (FPR) or system of spoken language. As a result of acquired deafness some children present with *deterioration* post-acquisition of a FPR. In most cases, pre-school profoundly deaf children will present with *delayed* acquisition of spoken language skills; some children may be classified as having *delayed* and *atypical* acquisition of spoken language skills. The term 'pre-verbal' is generally used to refer to the child who is using pre-recognisable spoken language patterns. The writer has found it useful, however, to consider deaf children who present with an established system of communication via sign language as *different*, i.e. a distinct group within the pre-verbal classification.

The need for uniform terminology and classification criteria, to facilitate the exchange of information and results, is acknowledged and remains of paramount importance. The paediatric IMPEVAL database used by implant programmes in the UK enables the professional to collect data along traditional lines. It also includes the classifications given in Table 11.4 which can be used to describe the child's communicative competence before and after implantation.

The terms 'pre-verbal', 'transitional' and 'functional' language are not linguistic terms in themselves, but they are used in a language-specific way. For example, they are used to describe a deaf child's ability in English, i.e. spoken language, *independently* from use of sign language or another spoken language if applicable. The effects of sensory impairment on language and cognitive development are complex and incorporate the long-standing debate on sign and spoken language systems. The principle that a systematic assessment of *verbal* communication skills involves more than performance-based assessments of listening

Table 11.4 Classification of linguistic status

Category 1 Preverbal

The deaf child functions at a pre-recognisable word level in a given language. The team professional must specify which language is being classified, for example English, Punjabi or British sign language-specific procedure

---

Category 2 Transitional

Recognisable word and phrase patterns are reported by the deaf child's family and known adults. It is possible to elicit some word phrase patterns in a familiar or closed-set context on a minimum of two occasions

---

Category 3 Functional language

The deaf child demonstrates the ability to use language(s) *spontaneously* and in a *systematic* way. For example, emerging speech patterns are used consistently in more than one context. A knowledge of meaning and syntactic rules is apparent. Equivalent features of language are noted in the case of a deaf child who uses sign language as the primary means of everyday communication.

---

and speaking skills in isolation still seems valid. Evaluation of the developing child's linguistic competence should include an investigation of the child's use of language, its content and form (Lahey, 1988). *Use* refers to the child's ability to use language in context, *content* represents the way the child conveys meaning, and *form* includes the surface aspects of language such as syntax, morphology and phonology.

To complete the classification with reliability a performance profile of five interrelated areas of investigation has been specified as shown in Table 11.5. All five areas are investigated when classifying a spoken language. The user may choose to use only the first three areas in the case of a sign language. The interrelationship of all areas is interpreted accordingly.

Table 11.5 Performance profile

Linguistic level	Area of investigation
1 Communication skills	Use of language,pragmatics, discourse skills, social skills
2 Receptive skills	Perception: auditory, visual, tactile mode, considerations Comprehension: semantics, syntax, lexis
3 Expressive skills	Expressive language (production): semantics, syntax, morphology, lexis. Mode considerations
4 Voice	Prosodic features or non-segmental aspects of speech
5 Speech	Speech skills: articulation and phonology

This performance profile was designed to enable an SLT to consider the linguistic level and the interrelationship of areas of investigation at a glance. Crystal (1992) advocates looking at the whole person and seeing his or her language system as a whole, including all the interactions among different levels of language structure. He states that phenomena at one level can influence those at another level. In the case of deaf children who use total communication, this will include monitoring changes in the child's reliance on sign language after implantation.

At the *receptive skills* level the relationship between traditional investigations of language comprehension and the less commonly investigated areas of perception and language modality is highlighted. It is important to recognise the distinction between auditory capacity and auditory performance. Profoundly deaf people need two things if auditory capacity is to be revealed in auditory performance – hearing aids and listening experiences (Boothroyd, 1993). The implication of this statement is that the team professional needs to look at emerging auditory skills in terms of the child's transition from demonstrable detection of auditory stimuli to his or her ability to listen without the help of lipreading in open-set language contexts and to use a telephone effectively. It is important to monitor the development of sound awareness at the non-linguistic level also, for example, the ability to detect and localise environmental sounds. A strong relationship between speech perception and speech production is reported in the literature. It may be useful to look at the role of audition after implantation, in the development, maintenance and prevention of deterioration in acquired speech skills in the case of children with acquired hearing loss.

At the *expressive skills* level, traditional investigations of vocabulary and syntax are extended to include investigations of language modality – at speech production, sign and written language levels, as appropriate.

It is important to look at emerging spoken language skills in terms of prosodic or non-segmental speech features at the *voice skills* level, as well as making traditional investigation of phonological and articulatory skills at the *speech level*. In the case of pre-verbal or low-verbal deaf children this should include careful documentation of the precursors of spoken language. It is useful to record information on the quantity, variety and quality of vocal patterns as well as emerging syllable structure before these children begin to use speech in a systematic way. The implant team SLT may wish to profile the development of diverse phonetic and phonological repertoires and to look at the rate of acquisition of spoken language skills after implantation.

The three profiles given in Tables 11.6 and 11.7 illustrate the potential use of a linguistic-based classification system over time. The findings are substantiated by performance measures and video analysis results at the agreed intervals.

Table 11.6 Classification of linguistic status: profiles

	Child A	Child B	Child C
Onset of deafness (years)	2;8	0	2;8
Age at implantation (years)	3;6	4;4	6;6
Duration of deafness (years)	10 months	4;4	3;10
Aetiology	Meningitis	Congenital	Meningitis

Child A

Although the duration between acquired profound deafness and cochlear implantation is less than 1 year, this child's profile demonstrates the acute deterioration in reportedly age-level communication skills which occurred before he received his implant. This child took approximately 18–24 months before he demonstrated consistent ability in performance-based tasks above a one-word level after implantation. Indirect reports and observations of the child showed lots of good signs in everyday communication from the 12-month interval. In this case speech skills show the most significant delay at the 24-month interval. By 48 months the child was described as intelligible to inexperienced listeners and also hearing peers in his mainstream school. Formal speech assessments suggest the characteristic errors and residual difficulties of a partially hearing child rather than a profoundly deaf child.

Child B

This example is of a child with profound deafness of congenital origin and more than 4 years' duration. An oral–aural mode of communication has always been used by the family and at school. Before implantation, this child presented with age-level interests and severe delay in all areas of communication in spite of the efforts and enthusiasm of her parents and teachers.

Characteristically, after implantation, the range of early communication skills and uses of language are the first to improve. By 6 months she had made demonstrable progress in expressive language and also voice skills. By 12 months she had learned to listen and carry out performance-based lipreading and listening tasks with reliability. Speech skills at the articulatory and phonological levels were delayed but improving. By 24 months she had been classified at the functional language stage and she continues to receive intensive help with receptive and expressive language as well as speech skills.

Child C

This child became deaf as a result of meningitis at 2;8 years. As with child A he is reported to have found it difficult to adjust to profound

Table 11.7 Classification: Preverbal (P), Transitional (T), Functional language (FL)

Interval	Level	Child A P	Child A T	Child A FL	Child B P	Child B T	Child B FL	Child C P	Child C T	Child C FL
Pre	1	•			•			•		
	2	•			•			•		
	3	•			•			•		
	4	•			•			•		
	5	•			•			•		
3 months	1	•				•		•		
	2	•			•			•		
	3	•			•			•		
	4	•			•			•		
	5	•			•			•		
6 months	1	•				•		•		
	2	•			•			•		
	3	•				•		•		
	4		•			•		•		
	5	•			•			•		
12 months	1		•				•		•	
	2		•		•			•		
	3		•		•			•		
	4		•		•				•	
	5	•			•			•		

TC at 18 months

Interval	Level	Child A P	Child A T	Child A FL	Child B P	Child B T	Child B FL	Child C P	Child C T	Child C FL
24 months	1			•			•		•	
	2		•			•			•	
	3			•		•			•	
	4			•		•			•	
	5		•			•		•		
36 months	1			•					•	
	2			•					•	
	3			•					•	
	4			•					•	
	5			•				•		

Linguistic level: (1) communication, (2) receptive, (3) expressive, (4) voice, and (5) speech bilateral deafness of sudden onset. At the time of implantation, this school-aged child relied on intuitive adults and peers in his everyday communication. He appeared to lack any knowledge of linguistic rules but like child B he presented with age-level interests and apparently intact non-verbal abilities. It was difficult to obtain a reliable estimate of his abilities and difficulties using performance measures. This profile illustrates characteristic slow change in receptive and production skills during the first 6 months after implantation. This child cooperated in a range of tasks with a low language level, but his responses were classed as inconsistent in all areas, excluding voice skills at that time. Audiological assessments after implantation demonstrated repeatable hearing sensitivity levels and this ability to detect speech may be reflected in the changes recorded in phonetic level speech features. In view of the child's educational needs, his age and the severity of overall linguistic delay, sign language was introduced approximately 18 months after implantation. By 24 months the child functioned at the transitional level in spoken language. By 36 months his spoken language skills without sign support remain at the transitional level.

Outline of a recommended speech–language assessment battery

Research findings now suggest that pre-verbal or low-verbal deaf children continue to make steady progress and may accelerate their rate of progress as late as 2 or even 3 years after implantation. The recommended assessment intervals for pre-school children in particular have already been described (Chapter 9). As a team SLT the author supports the view that, resources permitting, a comprehensive review by the implant programme should be offered to the implanted child's family after the 3-year follow-up programme, and at least at the fourth and fifth year interval.

It has been predicted that, in auditory terms, most implanted children are likely to present as potentially severely deaf or partially hearing children by the 3-year interval. The acquisition of receptive and expressive language skills will have started to follow a recognised sequence of development and a number of spoken language precursors will be in place. The implanted child's progress in speech and voice skills, however, may fall behind the rate of attainment at other linguistic levels. For this reason local professionals and parents may be eager for guidance on speech training from the team SLT at this stage. The 3- to 5-year interval after implantation may also be the most appropriate in terms of the pre-school implanted deaf child's readiness for formal speech intelligibility work.

During the first few years after implantation the nature of the child's learning crucially depends on how he or she organises what is heard and represents the input to him- or herself. The young hearing child learns to make links between what is heard and occurrences at the utterance level (Wanner and Gleitman, 1989). The importance of what is said to a child is far greater for a deaf child than for a hearing one (Wood et al., 1986). For similar reasons, Bench (1992) states that a performance-dominant assessment battery may fail to account for the intuitive characteristics of adult speech addressed to young deaf children. This is characterised by simplicity, consistency, redundancy and exaggerated prosody (Snow, 1972; Gleason, 1975; Nienhuys and Tikotin, 1985). A comprehensive speech and language assessment battery for young deaf children should include non-invasive measures of investigation such as video recordings of the child in different contexts and rating scales as well as performance-based procedures, some of which are illustrated in Table 11.8.

The SLT assessment battery has been designed so that a maximum of eight or nine procedures are required at a specified assessment interval. The choice is determined by the child's linguistic status, i.e. pre-verbal, transitional or functional language as already described.

PPECS (Pragmatics Profile of Early Communication Skills)

PPECS (Dewart and Summers, 1988) is an interview schedule used to establish a casework relationship and to ascertain the views of the family and local professionals on the preschool child's everyday communication strategies before implantation and at the 1-year and 3-year interval. Local practice suggests that PPECS also alerts the team SLT to any *mismatch* in perceptions of the child's overall linguistic competence as reported by family or local professionals.

NBC (Nursery Behaviour Checklist)

This observation profile (Nottingham Paediatric Cochlear Implant Programme, 1993) was designed to document actual early communication behaviours as observed in the child's everyday setting. It looks at the presence or absence of intentional behaviours, such as eye gaze, touching, bringing an object, pointing to self/object, any use of gesture or formal sign, exaggerated facial expression, gesture, and single utterance, gesture and continuous utterance, imitation of adult intonation patterns, and finally the use of consistent lip patterns or real word attempts. The NBC profile is based on observed rather than reported behaviours and is completed by a team SLT. It has been used with children aged from 2 up to 7 years usually in the early stages of the SLT outreach programme.

Table 11.8 Speech–language therapy: assessment battery

Linguistic levels*	Title	Origin	Type of test	Area of emphasis	Mode OA	TC
Level 1	Pragmatics Profile of Early Communication Skills	UK	Interview	Pragmatics, social skills	+	+
Level 1	Nursery Behaviour Checklist	UK	Pre-language rating scale	Early communication behaviours	+	+
Level 1, 2 & 3	Scales of Early Communication Skills	USA	Pre-school language scale	Verbal/non-verbal language	+	+
Level 2	Functional Lipreading and Lipreading Skills	UK	Informal profile/screening	Lipreading and listening skills	+	+
Level 2	Nucleus Perceptual Skills Assessment Battery	Europe	Test for area of deficit	Speech perception	+	+
Level 2	Test for Reception of Grammar (TROG)	UK	Test for area of deficit	Language comprehension	+	+
Level 3	South Tyneside Assessment of Syntactic Structures	UK	Test for area of deficit	Language syntax elicited	+	+
Level 4	Voice Skills Assessment	UK	Rating scale (recorded)	Prosody	+	
	Suprasegmental Assessment	USA	Rating scale	Prosody	+	
Level 5	Video (USA)	USA	Time sampling	Quantitative/qualitative analysis	+	
	Speech Intelligibility Rating (SIR)	UK	Rating scale	Analysis	+	
	PETAL Phonological Analysis Procedure	UK	Test for area of deficit	Phonology (hearing impairment)	+	
	Edinburgh Articulation Test	UK	Test for area of deficit	Articulation	+	
	Phonological Assessment of Child's Speech	UK	Test for area of deficit	Phonological processes	+	

*Linguistic level: (1) communication; (2) receptive; (3) expressive; (4) voice and (5) speech.

SECS (Scales of Early Communication Skills for Hearing Impaired Children)

The detailed criteria and examples which accompany this scale (Moog and Geers, 1975), devised at the Central Institute for the Deaf (USA), appear to ensure greater inter-user reliability than is normally achieved with rating scales. Information on early receptive, expressive and non-verbal language skills is provided in a user-friendly format. The results are accessible to non-SLT and non-teaching support staff and to the child's family, after discussion.

FLLS (Functional Lipreading and Listening Skills)

The FLLS profile (Nottingham Paediatric Cochlear Implant Programme, 1993) (Table 11.9) was designed to investigate emerging lipreading and listening skills at a one-word level and later at a sentence level, using real objects and picture-related materials, e.g. the Real Objects Subtest of the Derbyshire Language Scheme (Knowles and Masidlover, 1982). It is used with children at the transitional and functional language level of linguistic ability from around 3 years of age.

The illustration demonstrates a child's developing listening skills using the Bamford, Köwal and Bench (BKB) picture-related sentence lists (Bench and Bamford, 1979). The child was classified as preverbal at the time of implantation. This type of profile demonstrates the initial reliance on lipreading and listening. By 30 months good progress is noted in sentence level tasks and more rapid progress occurs between 30 and 36 months, when the child begins to achieve high level scores in closed set tasks using listening alone.

Table 11.9 Functional lipreading and listening skills (FLLS)

Date and audio information	WLR	LR	X2	Wr	TC	NR
Pre-implant	CNT	CNT				
12 months post-implant	CNT	CNT				
24 months post-implant BKB PR List 1	CNT	7	6		1	2
30 months post-implant BKB PR List 4		14	2			
36 months post-implant BKB PR List 6	13	2	1			

BKB PR = Bamford, Köwal and Bench Picture Related Sentence Lists. WLR= without lipreading; L2 = lipreading; X2 = repetition; Wr = written cue; TC = total communication; NR = no response; CNT = could not test.

It is possible to make more than one entry in the profile at a speci-fied assessment interval. The FLLS is administered using live voice and generally in the child's everyday home or school setting. It provides useful information on whether the young implanted child is ready to carry out a recorded speech test of hearing in a clinic setting.

NPSAB (Nucleus Perceptual Skills Assessment Battery (TAPS))

This assessment battery is known as TAPS (Reid and Lennhardt, 1993). It was designed by Cochlear AG to look at the perceptual skills of chil-dren between the ages of 2 and 15 years. A common set of research based measures known as the Test of Auditory Perception of Speech (TAPS) has been adapted for use with English, French and German-speaking children as follows.

Category 1

This category assesses the child's awareness of speech sounds (pres-ence or absence) using auditory cues alone.

Category 2

This category assesses the child's ability to differentiate between seg-mental features using durational and intensity cues via auditory cues alone.

Category 3

This category assesses the child's ability to identify speech terms by dif-ferentiating spectral information via auditory cues alone.

Category 4

This category assesses the child's ability to identify the word stimulus from a group of three words, two of which are visually homophonous, using auditory–visual cues.

Category 5

This category assesses the child's ability to recognise speech related to a particular topic in a modified open set format using auditory cues alone. A production level response is required in category five (Reid and Lennhardt, 1993).

At the time of writing approximately 75% of the implanted children in the Nottingham Programme can complete part or all of the TAPS battery between the 12- and 24-month interval. Deaf children at the more than two-word level of language comprehension and production may achieve reliable results on categories 1, 2 and 3 within the first 12 months of implantation. Until now confident results on the modified open-set tasks in category 5 are rarely recorded before the 18–24 month interval in the case of pre-school implanted children.

TROG (Test for Reception of Grammar)

The Test for Reception of Grammar (TROG – Bishop, 1989) is a multiple choice test of language comprehension which consists of 80 four-choice items. The test is appropriate for a wide age range of 4–12 years. It has been standardised on a UK population and includes some normative data on adults. No expressive speech is required from the subject in this test. Picture and vocabulary stimuli have been selected to ensure low ambiguity and the control of non-linguistic factors such as plausibility. In the case of deaf children it is useful to record additional information on mode of presentation, audition or audition plus vision, and to make a note of any modifications required, for example, repetition. The test results may be interpreted quantitatively and also qualitatively. The SLT may wish to investigate whether the child's errors are predominantly lexical or grammatical. TROG results may be compared with the findings obtained on other comprehension tests, notably the British Picture Vocabulary scale (Dunn, Dunn, Whetton and Pintilie, 1982). This test enables the assessor to compare the implanted deaf child's performance with that of his or her hearing peers.

STASS (South Tyneside Assessment of Syntactic Structures)

This picture-related screening procedure (Armstrong and Ainley, 1986) had been designed to assess the language ability of children at the expressive syntax level. It is based on the Language Assessment Remediation and Screening Procedure (LARSP) developed by Crystal et al. (1989). Specialised SLTs within the UK use an agreed code of modifications to transcribe the profoundly deaf child's language production at the non-speech as well as the speech level.

STASS provides a useful baseline measure in the case of sign-dominant deaf children. It has also been found useful with older deaf children from 7 to 10 years who function at a low verbal level of ability. It is rarely used by the Nottingham team SLTs before the 12-month interval.

The next seven procedures have been selected to investigate and describe the development of spoken language at several distinct but interrelated levels. Objective measurements of speech skills which involve listeners' judgements of recorded speech samples or analysis of speech production using computer-based visual displays may of necessity be a deferred aim when working with preschool deaf children. The absence of robust assessment procedures for low verbal deaf children has been reported by SLTs and other professionals who wish to look at emerging spoken language skills. Nevertheless it is suggested that careful documentation of emerging skills at the production level, i.e. the acquisition of actual rather than predicted speech patterns after implantation, by a team SLT is an extremely worth-while aim in itself. The diversity of individual children's phonetic and phonological repertoires continues to confound the expectation of many professionals associated with cochlear implantation.

VSA (Voice Skills Assessment Battery)

For the reasons just given a rating scale was devised by the Nottingham SLTs to look at a range of prosodic or voice features as used by the implanted children in everyday settings. The VSA (Nottingham Paediatric Cochlear Implant Programme, 1993) can also be used as part of video sample analysis procedures to highlight specific prosodic strengths or difficulties. The details of this rating scale are given in Table 11.10.

Table 11.10 Voice skills assessment rating scale

Airstream:	Control established ☐	Overall problem ☐	Segmental errors ☐
Voice quality:	Normal ☐ Whisper ☐	Breathy ☐	Tense ☐ Creaky ☐
Pitch range:	Normal ☐	Too wide ☐	Too narrow ☐
Pitch control:	Established ☐	Fluctuating ☐	
Pitch variability: normal	High versus restricted ☐ Drifts up at end of sentence ☐	Monotonous ☐	Drifts down at end of sentence ☐
Loudness:	Control established ☐	Poor control ☐	
Rate of delivery:	Normal ☐	Too fast ☐	Too slow ☐
Resonance:	Acceptable ☐	Hypernasal ☐	Hyponasal ☐ Segmental errors ☐
Rhythm:	Stress timing ☐ Sound timing ☐	Syllable timing ☐	Word timing ☐
Intonation:	Full set of English contrasts ☐ Contrast by altering length ☐	Contrast absent/or stereotype pattern ☐ Contrast by altering loudness ☐	

CID Phonetic Inventory: suprasegmental aspects

The initial section of this well-known assessment (Moog, 1988) has been used successfully to provide time-effective and useful information on implanted children with transitional or functional language level abilities.

At the time of writing, the author's group have begun to use the Fundamental Speech Skills Test (FSST – Levitt, Youdelman and Head, 1990) with implanted deaf children who are ready to carry out a performance-based test with reliability. As an SLT the author welcomes the emphasis of the FSST on the basic aspects of speech production: breath stream capacity; elementary articulation; pitch control; syllabification; stress; and intonation contours. In spite of some minor administration difficulties caused by apparent differences between American English and British English, the opportunity to compare an individual child's FSST performance profile with other non-implanted students who have a similar hearing loss is welcome. The current FSST normative population is American which must be remembered by test users in other countries.

Video analysis of running speech (USA)

This is a time-sampling method of analysis using video recordings of the deaf child's speech and the procedure has been described by Osberger and colleagues (Osberger, 1989; Osberger et al., 1991). It enables the clinician, usually an SLT, to make a comparison of the child's speech within child over time and across children using different cochlear implants, tactile or hearing aids. The initial profile looks at the low-verbal deaf child's utterances in terms of speech, speech-like, non-speech and other patterns. A choice of three analytical procedures – a consonant and vowel summary, a summary for place of a articulation and a place–voice–manner error pattern analysis – can be made once the initial profile has been completed. The original procedure has been adapted for users in the UK using the existing consonant system and an adapted vowel system based on Moore (1989). It is known as PASS (Profile of Actual Speech Skills).

Experience in Nottingham suggests that this profile provides invaluable information on the changing status of speech and voice skills during the first year after implantation, and thereafter in cases where children are not linguistically ready to complete a formal test of speech skills. It is usually not suitable for prospective implant candidates who have established speech skills.

SIR (Speech Intelligibility Rating)

Intelligibility is a function of the skills of listener and speaker and so intelligibility ratings or summaries are relative not absolute (Parker and

Irlam, 1994). The purpose of the SIR rating scale (Nottingham Paediatric Cochlear Implant Programme, 1993) is to document emerging voice skills based on recorded and live assessment outcomes. The current six categories have been adapted from previous work on the speech intelligibility of adult deaf speakers by Parker and others. It is planned to adapt and evaluate the outlined criteria using independent listeners and visual display measurements once a larger group of implanted children has become available. The categories are outlined in Table 11.11.

Table 11.11 Speech intelligibility rating (SIR)

Category	Speech Intelligibility Rating
6	Speech intelligible to all listeners
5	Speech intelligible to listeners with little experience of the speech of a deaf speaker
4	Speech intelligible to a listener who concentrates and lipreads
3	Speech unintelligible. Experienced listeners can follow a known topic via lipreading and context cues. It is not possible to follow an audio-tape sample
2	The primary mode of communication is manual. The speech or vocalisation patterns which accompany the use of sign/ gesture may give some additional information at the lipreading level
1	Pre-recognisable words in spoken language

PETAL (speech assessment procedure)

PETAL is a comprehensive speech assessment procedure which is being developed for use with deaf children and adults by A. Parker, A.B. King and R. Wright (unpublished data). It promotes the use of a phonological therapy approach of assessment and management as originally described by Grunwell (1987) and also by Dean et al. (1990):

- Phonological therapy should be systematically planned and based on an analysis of speech output.
- Treatment should be essentially concerned with widening the range of sound contrasts available to the child in a variety of contexts. The emphasis should be on changing sound patterns rather than teaching individual sounds.

As well as investigating the deaf child's speech at a single-word level, PETAL also investigates the child's vowel and diphthong system, ability to use consonant sounds contrastively, intonation and overall intelligibility in recorded samples of target words, for example, counting, days of the week or other appropriate words and phrases with a low language load. The school-aged deaf child may also be recorded reading and re-telling a story in his or her own words as well as having a 'chat' with the assessor or interactor.

It is important to look at the child's full phonological system and not just the phonetic inventory. The SLT should also note the incidence of non-English sounds, the use of homonyms, and the effects of co-articulation on the variable production of sounds as well as words.

EAT (Edinburgh Articulation Test)

The EAT (Anthony et al., 1971) is a conventional articulation test familiar to professionals in the UK. It enables a comparison of findings to be made between a deaf speaker and a hearing peer. The aim of this test is to provide a sensitive and economical instrument for looking at the spoken language of very young children. It is concerned only with consonant articulations. No attention is given to vowels, rhythm, intonation or voice quality (Abercrombie, 1971). The limitations of the quantitative analysis of the EAT are self-evident when working with profoundly deaf speakers. The qualitative analysis, however, appears to provide a useful guideline to changes in speech patterns over a 2- to 3-year interval. The implanted child's speech production can be recorded under one of six categories: adult form; minor variations; almost mature; immature; very immature; and atypical. The resulting EAT profile provides information for non-SLTs in an accessible format. This procedure has been found most useful with deaf children who have established language and those who have become deaf once language is established.

PACS (Phonological Assessment of Child's Speech)

The PACS phonological analyses procedure was first described by Grunwell (1985). It aims to look at the presence or absence of phonological processes at both the structural and systemic levels of speech and is outlined in Table 11.12.

It should be remembered that PACS has been devised to look at speech processes in the hearing population. Although it is time-consuming to administer and interpret, experience suggests that its use enables an implant team SLT to provide clear and appropriate speech goals to the child's family and local professionals. PACS is administered by the Nottingham SLTs once, at the 3-year interval, to those children at or near age-level linguistic skills, or sooner in the case of children with acquired hearing loss.

An SLT assessment battery profile of a young low verbal deaf child is given in Table 11.13.

Factors influencing rate of progress

As with tactile and acoustic hearing aid users, the form or level of training provided to implanted children may be an important variable in

Table 11.12 Phonological Asessment of Child's Speech (PACS)*

Structural simplifications	Systemic simplifications
Weak syllable deletion	Fronting
Final consonant deletion	Stopping
Vocalisation of syllabic lateral	Gliding of liquids
Cluster reduction	De-nasalisation
Extraneous elements	Backing
Epenthesis	Palatising
Metathesis	Glottalising
Context-sensitive voicing	Gliding of liquids
Consonant harmony	Labialisation
Reduplication	Other

*Grunwell (1985).

determining the type of communication skills they ultimately acquire (Alcántara et al., 1990). Along with other team professionals, a team SLT aims not only to develop a set of basic perceptual skills but also to establish a set of basic motor skills at the speech production level. The long-term aims for the child are: to develop and consolidate the capacity for speech memory and recall of speech patterns after direct training has been removed; to develop the ability to transfer trained speech skills on to new contexts; and, finally, to generate higher level linguistic processing and production skills from the everyday environment.

Some useful principles of planning individual remediation programmes using a structural analysis approach have been outlined by Lund and Duchan (1988) as follows: first, careful observation to determine what the child is attempting and the specific problems the child is having in everyday communication; second, to establish meaningful goals for the child we need to know the discrepancies between what the child is intending to communicate and what is actually being communicated; third, in judging the efficacy of therapy we must be aware that varying language behaviours are displayed in different contexts. By implication, a structural analysis approach as outlined is an ongoing assessment approach. It does not stop when therapy begins. Such a perspective enables the professional to identify what is being attempted by the child, what is being accomplished and what conditions promote or impede success. In the literature it is suggested that normal hearing children need to be exposed to language before the age of 3 years for them to develop a language system effortlessly (Tyler and Fryauf-Bertschy, 1992). In the deafness management quotient (DMQ), Northern and Downs (1978) outlined the five factors of residual hearing, central intactness, intellectual factors, family constellation and socioeconomic status as contributing to the deaf child's ultimate progress. In the Social Language Predictor Index (SLPI), Geers and Moog (1987) investigated the effects of residual hearing capacity,

Table 11.13 Speech and language assessment IMPEVAL database record

Name of procedure	Linguistic category	Assessment interval (months) pre-implant					
		(P)	3 P	6 P	12 FL	24 FL	36 FL
Interview (PPECS)	P T FL	✓	–	–	✓	–	✓
Speech Intelligibility Rating (SIR)	P T FL	✓	✓	✓	✓	✓	✓
Voice Skills Assessment (VSA)	P T FL	CNT	✓	–	✓	✓	✓
Nursery Behaviour Checklist	P T –	✓	*	*	✓	–	–
Video Analysis: Osberger	P T –	✓	✓	✓	✓	✓	–
Conversation Skills Profile	– – FL	CNT	CNT	CNT	CNT	✓	✓
Scales of Early Communication Skills (SECS)	P T FL	*	*	*	✓	✓	✓
Edinburgh Articulation Test (EAT)	– T FL	CNT	CNT	CNT	✓	✓	✓
Speech Assessment Procedure (SAP)	– T FL	CNT	CNT	CNT	✓	✓	✓
Suprasegmental Assessment (CID)	– T FL	CNT	CNT	CNT	CNT	✓	✓
Functional Listening Skills (FLS)	– T FL	CNT	CNT	CNT	*	✓	✓
Nucleus Perceptual Skills Assessment Battery (TAPS)	– T FL	–	–	–	*	*	–
Elicited Syntax Assessment (STASS)	– T FL	CNT	–	CNT	CNT	✓	✓
Test for Reception of Grammar (TROG)	– – FL	CNT	–	–	CNT	*	✓
Phonological Assessment of child Speech (PACS)	– – FL	–	–	–	–	–	✓

CNT, could not test; *, recommended; –, not appropriate. P, pre-verbal: T, transitional; FL, functional language.

language competence, non-verbal intelligence, family support and the child's speech communication attitude on the eventual speech prognosis of the profoundly deaf child.

The following priority areas of investigation have been identified as part of a detailed study of the development of spoken language skills after cochlear implantation Dyar, (1992):

Communication skills:	Uses of language, conversation and social skills
Speech:	Motor skills development; encoding skills at phonetic and phonological levels
Voice:	The development of prosodic skills at structural and systemic levels
Receptive skills:	The rate of development of listening skills in relation to auditory acuity; perceptual/mode dominance at auditory and visual levels; the development of language comprehension in terms of vocabulary, meaning and syntax
Expressive skills:	Processing abilities at speech, sign and written language levels; the development of expressive language in terms of vocabulary meaning and syntax
Everyday communication:	Investigation of attitudes to communication and styles of interaction as well as expectation levels after implantation
IQ and 3 Rs:	Non-verbal IQ; academic attainments; child's attitude to work
Social needs:	Investigation of the age-appropriate social opportunities outside of school/home
Emotional development:	Investigation of the deaf or deafened child's ability to show affect in appropriate ways
Personality:	Investigation of the child's self-image, coping strategies and learning style
Friendships:	Ability to make friends with other deaf and hearing children current/future peers
Levels of support:	Amount and nature of specialist support at the local level

A team SLT may also need to investigate communication and language difficulties which result from non-deafness-related causes, especially in a small number of cases where the implanted child fails to develop listening and speech skills at the expected rate of development inspite of good auditory sensitivity levels after implantation.

Professionals should not be trying to fit children to schools but working out individual arrangements best suited to each child (Webster and Ellwood, 1986). The decision about selecting the most appropriate educational setting for the young implanted child remains difficult for many families. McCracken and Sutherland (1991) give the following guidelines: parents/families should consider the current and predicted development of their child's language and speech; they should consider the child's potential ability to convey his or her everyday needs independently, the personality of their child, the child's general mental ability – insofar as it can be ascertained, and whether their child has additional special educational needs apart from deafness. Having highlighted a range of contributing factors, ultimately it is the child who must decide the pace of progress after implantation.

Future trends issues and concerns

How the introduction of auditory information through the cochlear implant affects cognitive processes and, in turn, language for hearing-impaired children is an area worthy of investigation (Hasenstab, 1993). This statement implies that initial and subsequent changes in implant device settings may result in subtle changes in an implanted child's behaviour and communication skills. It seems important therefore to discuss when and why changes to device settings are made, at an inter-disciplinary level. This will enable implant programmes to conduct studies of control groups or equivalent children rather than random control trials (Haggard, 1992).

Established links with other paediatric implant programmes suggest that team SLTs would support more uniform assessment protocols and greater agreement about recommended assessment intervals at an inter-team level. In the case of pre-verbal deaf children guidance is constantly being sought on how to decide whether hearing aids have been worn for a sufficient length of time and with reliability. Deaf children with additional or complex needs continue to challenge our abilities to assess the child's cognitive, linguistic and motor skills. A critical need continues to exist for studies producing standardised testing instruments, establishing normative data for children of various ages with varying levels of hearing impairment (Tobey, 1993). Norm-referenced tests, for example, the Fundamental Speech Skills Test (FSST), need to be validated and standardised on a large population of severe and profoundly deaf children, as an extension of the available normative data. At the time of writing SLTs and educators are beginning to request help with frameworks of assessment for higher-level linguistic skills as pre-school-implanted deaf children progress beyond the subject–verb–object level, but are not yet ready to complete time-consuming formal speech perception assessment batteries. The adaptation of child-appropriate speech perception measures and the search for linguistically 'equivalent' vocabulary and sentence patterns across more than one spoken language (Reid and Lennhardt, 1993) are, in spite of inherent difficulties, a welcome trend in this area.

The assessment of pragmatic–linguistics, such as the use of language and discourse or conversation strategies in spoken language by profoundly deaf children, has become increasingly important with the advent of cochlear implants. Clinical sociolinguistics is perhaps a less developed area (Ball, 1992). The professional with an interest in socio-linguistics looks at the interaction of the child in relation to class membership, sex, regional background, ethnic background, age and the use of language varieties. It may also encompass the study of bilingualism. Most SLTs who have chosen to specialise in hearing impairment have a particular interest in bilingualism; the role of sign language and the need to evaluate the shift in language dominance between sign language and spoken language after implantation seems an important issue to look at, especially in those children who are classified as 'sign dominant' before implantation.

The literature on linguistic outcomes which result from those implanted children who were in the linguistically developing stage at the time of implantation remains sparse (Ruben, 1992). Ruben also reminds us that the essential purpose of the intervention in the linguistically developing child is to enable the child to develop optimal language. Finally, the importance of reporting individual scores is emphasised by Tyler (1993). He states that reporting average scores across individuals does not specify the most critical information. It can also be misleading to report the percentage of children scoring above chance before and after surgery; it fails to indicate the magnitude of the pre- and postoperative differences. What is important is the absolute level of performance for each child. For this reason a solution may be to show individual data in scattergrams or bar graphs. As well as reporting reasons for device failure, implant team professionals need to investigate and share information on potential reasons for poor performance in those children who appear to be 'under-functioning' as well as providing results on star implant users.

Conclusion

In recent years the traditional view of SLTs 'correcting' children's speech on weekly visits to an outpatient's clinic has become an outmoded one (Webster and Wood, 1989). Webster and Wood continue by stating that SLTs can make significant contributions to the overall management of communication. This may include handing on skills and strategies to those who have day-to-day contact with hearing-impaired children, as described earlier in this chapter.

As an implant team-based SLT, the author supports the view that the assessment of very young children necessitates the development of specific measures rather than adapting those of an adult programme (Archbold, 1992). The philosophy of the Nottingham programme is that changes in social adjustment, communication skills and educational attainments should be monitored by professionals with experience of this age group. The dilemma of choosing an analytical, synthetic or combined approach to rehabilitation and training is not a critical issue when supporting pre-school profoundly deaf children with conventional acoustic aids, tactile aids or cochlear implants. What is needed is initially to look at the actual rather than predicted outcomes, especially with pre-verbal or low-verbal deaf children who are not ready to carry out performance-based test measures.

Haggard (1991) argued for robust exportable rehabilitation methods so that local rehabilitation personnel may continue the work started by the implant team with continuity of methods. It is hoped that this view has been reflected in the description of the SLT assessment battery, and the outreach visits and activities which may be undertaken by an implant team SLT.

As a clinician who has chosen to work exclusively with deaf children, the writer finds it necessary constantly to revise her expectations and appraise the impact of profound deafness of congenital or acquired origin in light of new technology. Association with a paediatric cochlear implant programme has rekindled her respect for the phenomenal role of audition in the acquisition of effective everyday spoken language skills.

References

Abercrombie, J. (1971). In A. Anthony, D. Bogle, T. Ingram and M. McIsaac (eds), *The Edinburgh Articulation Test*. Edinburgh: Churchill Livingstone.

Alcántara, J.I., Whitford, L.A., Blamey, P.J., Cowan, R.S.C. and Clark, G. M. (1990). Tactile feature recognition by deaf children. *Journal of the Acoustical Society of America*, **88** (3), 1260–1274.

Anthony, A., Bogle, D., Ingram, T. and McIsaac, M. (eds) (1971). *The Edinburgh Articulation Test*. Edinburgh: Churchill Livingstone.

Archbold, S.M. (1992). The development of a paediatric cochlear implant programme: A case study. *Journal of the British Association Teachers of the Deaf*, **16** (1), 17–26.

Armstrong, S. and Ainley, M. (1986). *STASS: South Tyneside Assessment of Syntactic Structures*. Northumberland: STASS Publications.

Ball, M. (1992). *Clinician's Guide to Linguistic Profiling of Language Impairment*. Kibworth: Far Communications.

Bench, J. (1992). *Communication skills in Hearing Impaired Children*. London: Whurr.

Bench, J. and Bamford, J. (1979). *Speech–Hearing Tests and the Spoken Language of Hearing Impaired Children*. London: Academic Press.

Bishop, D.V.M. (1989). *Test for Reception of Grammar*, 2nd edn. Available from the author, MRC Applied Psychology Unit, 15 Chaucer Road, Cambridge.

Bloom, J. and Lahey, M. (1978). *Language Development and Language Disorders*. New York: John Wiley.

Bloomfield, L. (1933). *Language*. New York: Henry Holt, 1961.

Boothroyd, A. (1993). Profound deafness. In R.S. Tyler (ed.), *Cochlear Implants: Audiological Foundations*. London: Whurr.

Chomsky, N. (1965). *Aspects of the Theory of Syntax*. Cambridge, MA: MIT press.

Crystal, D. (1992). *Profiling Linguistic Disability*, 2nd edn. London: Whurr.

Crystal, D., Fletcher, P. and Garman, M. (1989). Language Assessment, Remediation and Screening Procedure (LARSP). In *Grammatical Analysis of Language Disability*, 2nd edn. London: Whurr.

Dean, E., Howell, J., Hill, A. and Waters, D. (1990). *Metaphon Resource Pack*. Windsor: NFER-Nelson.

Dewart, H. and Summers, S. (1988). *Pragmatics Profile of Early Communication Skills*. Windsor: NFER-Nelson.

Dunn, L.M., Dunn, L.M., Whetton, C. and Pintilie, D. (1982). *British Picture Vocabulary Scale*. Windsor: NFER-Nelson.

Dyar, D. (1992). The development of spoken language skills after cochlear implantation: results obtained from one child during a 0–3 year interval. Presentation at The First European Symposium on Paediatric Cochlear Implantation, Nottingham, 1992.

Dyson, S. (1987). Reasons for assessment rhetoric and reality in the assessment of children with disabilities. In T. Booth and W. Swann (eds), *Including Pupils with Disabilities*. Milton Keynes: Open University Press.

Geers, A. and Moog, J. (1987). Predicting spoken language acquisition of profoundly impaired children. *Journal of Speech and Hearing Disorders*, 2, 84–94.

Gleason, J.B. (1975). Fathers and other strangers: mens speech to young children. In D.F. Dato (ed.), *Development Linguistics: Theories and Applications*. Washington DC: Georgetown University Press.

Grunwell, P. (1985). *Phonological Assessment of Child Speech (PACS)*. Windsor: NFER-Nelson.

Grunwell, P. (1987). *Clinical Phonology*, 2nd edn. London: Croom Helm.

Haggard, M. (1991). Introduction: Cochlear implants in perspective. In H. Cooper, (ed.), *Cochlear Implants: A Practical Guide*, London: Whurr.

Haggard, M. (1992). Health economics aspects of paediatric cochlear implantation. Keynote address: First European Symposium on Paediatric Cochlear Implantation, Nottingham, September 1992.

Hasenstab, S. (1993). Cognitive and linguistic changes in children using Nucleus multichannel cochlear implants. Proceedings of the Third International Cochlear Implant Conference, Innsbruck, Austria, April 1993.

Haynes, C. (1989). Language development in the school years – what can go wrong? In K. Mogford and J. Sadler (eds), *Child Language Disability: Implications in an Educational Setting*. Clevedon: Multilingual Matters.

Knowles, W. and Masidlover, M. (1982). *Derbyshire Language Scheme*. Derbyshire County Council.

Lahey, M. (1988). *Language Disorders and Language Development*. New York: Macmillan.

Laurenzi, C. (1993). The bionic ear and the mythology of paediatric implants. *British Journal of Audiology*, 27, 1–5.

Levitt, H., Youdelman, K. and Head, J. (1990). *Fundamental Speech Skills Test*. Obtain from Cochlear Corporation, 61 Inverness Drive East, Suite 200, Englewood, Colorado, USA.

Lund, N. and Duchan, J. (1988). *Assessing Children, Language in Naturalistic Contexts*. Englewood Cliffs, NJ: Prentice Hall.

Luterman, D. (1987). *Deafness in the Family*. San Diego, CA: College-Hill Press.

McCracken, W. and Sutherland, H. (1991). Deaf ability not disability. *A Guide for Parents of Hearing Impaired Children*. Clevedon: Multilingual Matters.

Moog, J. (1988). *CID Phonetic Inventory*. St Louis, USA: Central Institute for the Deaf.

Moog, J. and Geers, A. (1975). *Scales of Early Communication Skills for Hearing Impaired Children*. St Louis, USA: Central Institute for the Deaf.

Moore, B.C.J. (1989). *Introduction to the Psychology of Hearing*, 3rd Edn. London: Academic Press.

Nienhuys, T.G. and Tikotim, J.A. (1985). Mother–infant interaction: pre-speech communication in hearing and deaf babies. *Australian Journal of Teacher of the Deaf*, **26**, 4–12.

Nottingham Paediatric Cochlear Implant Programme (1993). *Cochlear Implant Evaluation Database – Speech and Language Therapy Protocols*, Nottingham, UK.

Northern, J. and Downs, M. (eds) (1978). Deafness Management Quotient (DMQ). In *Hearing in Children*. Baltimore, MA: Williams & Wilkins.

Osberger, M.J. (1989). Speech production in profoundly hearing impaired children with reference to cochlear implants. In E. Owens and D. Kessler (eds), *Cochlear Implants in Young Deaf Children*. Boston: College-Hill Press.

Osberger, M.J., Robbins, A.M., Berry, S.W., Todd, L., Hesketh, L.J. and Sedey, A. (1991). Analysis of spontaneous speech samples of children with a cochlear implant or tactile aid. *American Journal of Otology*, **12** (Suppl.), 151–164.

Parker, A. and Irlam, S. (1994). Intelligibility and deafness: the skills of listener and speaker. In Wirz, S.L. (ed.), *Perceptual Approaches to Speech and Language Disorders*, in press. London: Whurr.

Reid, J. and Lennhardt, M. (1993). Speech perception test results for European children using the Nucleus cochlear implant. Presentation at Third International Cochlear Implant Conference, Innsbruck, Austria, April 1993.

Ruben, R.J. (1992). The paediatric cochlear implant. Keynote address: First European Symposium on Paediatric Cochlear Implantation, Nottingham, UK, September 1992.

Snow, C.E. (1972). Mother's speech to children learning language. *Child Development*, **43**, 549–565.

Tobey, E.A. (1993). Speech production. In R.S. Tyler (ed.), *Cochlear Implants: Audiological Foundations*. London: Whurr.

Tyler, R.S. (1993). Speech perception by children. In Tyler, R.S. (ed.), *Cochlear Implants: Audiological Foundations*. London: Whurr.

Tyler, R.S. and Fryauf-Bertschy, H. (1992). Hearing abilities of children with cochlear implants. In N. Tye-Murray (ed.), *Cochlear Implants for Children: A Handbook for Parents, Teachers, Speech and Hearing Professionals*. Washington DC: Alexander Graham Bell Association for the Deaf.

Wanner, E. and Gleitman, L. (1989). *Language Acquisition: The State of the Art*. Cambridge: Cambridge University Press.

Webster, A. and Elwood, J. (1986). *The Hearing Impaired Child in the Ordinary School*. London: Croom-Helm.

Webster, A. and Wood, D. (1989). *Special Needs in Ordinary Schools: Children with Hearing Difficulties*. London: Cassell Education.

Wood, D., Wood, H., Griffith, A. and Howarth, I. (1986). *Teaching and Talking with Deaf Children*. Chichester: John Wiley & Sons.

Chapter 12
Family perspectives

HAZEL LLOYD

Throughout the book, emphasis on the importance of the role of the child's family during the process of implantation has been stressed. This chapter gives parents the opportunity to express some of their thoughts and feelings in their own words. Some contributions are taken from parents' diaries, some from articles written for our newsletter and others from responses to questionnaires. To protect the children and their families all names have been changed.

Parents' use of diaries

In the Nottingham Programme we have found parents' diaries to be extremely useful. As many of our children live a great distance away, often several hundred miles, it is not possible to 'drop in when passing' to see how the child and family are getting along. Naturally, if there is any cause for concern we encourage parents or local professionals to telephone us. However, as visits to the child's home and school are only once a month in the first year and bi-monthly in the second and third years, it is not only necessary, but also extremely helpful to us, if we can be made aware of what has taken place (or not taken place), while we are not around. To ensure that parents are fully aware of what is expected of them, information on how to use the diary is included as shown below.

We are interested to know:

- How the child reacts to wearing the processor, in the home situation
- Does he like it?
- How long does he wear it for?
- Have there been any problems getting him to wear it?
- Are there any differences in his behaviour, when he is wearing it, for example, with family or strangers?

We also need to monitor the development of his listening skills:

- Have you noticed responses to sounds?
- Positive reactions to sounds?
- Negative reactions to sound?
- Any sign of looking in the direction of sound?
- Any sign of being able to distinguish one sound from another?

We also need to monitor any change in communication when wearing the processor:

- Have you noticed changes in vocalisation? In quantity or quality?
- Imitation of sounds?
- Changes in listening or looking in conversation?
- Changes in language or vocabulary use?

These points are discussed at length when the parents are first given their diaries.

The format used by the parents for their diaries varies immensely. One mother reported that she found writing the diary at the end of each day quite therapeutic. She wrote not only about what her child had done throughout the day, but also commented on her feelings at the time, sometimes of joy, but at other times of frustration and anger, saying that somehow writing it all down helped. Other busy parents found that writing the most profound comment of the day was the most useful format for them. Whatever the style or format, both my colleagues and I have found their comments invaluable in helping to monitor each individual child's progress.

Parents too have found their own diaries useful, especially at times when their child appears to be making very little progress. Looking back through their diaries to previous months or years helps them to focus their concerns realistically, often making them aware just how far their child has progressed and often giving them impetus to work harder and at the same time be patient, particularly with a very young child.

Making the decision

Embarking on the journey of cochlear implantation with a young son or daughter is not an easy road to take and can be fraught with many trials and tribulations, not least of which involves making the initial decision. For many parents this would have been extremely traumatic, and in the early years many encountered opposition from many quarters. At no point during the entire assessment period, which may take many months, should parents be pressured regarding their final decision. Parents should be encouraged to talk to as many people as possible, including families who already have an implanted child, but also to families who feel that implantation is not the way forward for their child. It is most important that each family is satisfied that they have explored all avenues before making an informed decision for their deaf child.

Carol's father reported talking to his daughter's headmistress, who was a confirmed supporter of British Sign Language and of the deaf community. The headmistress asked him numerous questions about the decision he and his wife were about to make, to allow their daughter to have a cochlear implant. After several hours of deep discussion, many disagreements and some agreement, the headmistress finally commented that, although she personally did not agree with cochlear implants for young children, she felt that she had given the father a thorough interrogation into his reasons for making the decision and that he was justified in saying that his decision was well informed. She then confirmed that the child's school would do whatever was necessary to help make sure the cochlear implant was successful.

Making the decision on behalf of a young child, without the child's real knowledge or understanding of what is to happen to him or her, is perhaps what makes the decision so difficult to make. For Tom's parents, making the decision to allow their 3-year-old son to have a cochlear implant was to give their son a choice in later life. They wrote:

> Our son is a healthy, robust, happy, deaf, young man. He uses Sign Supported English to make his needs known to us, and we talk and sign to him. He was born hearing and suffered with meningitis at the age of two years, when he lost his hearing completely. After wearing high-powered hearing aids for two years, with no apparent benefit we decided to find out if he was a suitable candidate for a cochlear implant. Why did we feel a cochlear implant would be appropriate for our son? Because we wanted to give him a choice later in life. As our son is using sign language, and attends a unit where he is taught using Sign Supported English, we know that he will always have this facility of communication available to him. However, we also wanted to give him the opportunity to be part of the hearing community, hence a cochlear implant. If in later life, after using the implant consistently throughout his learning years, he chooses to only be part of the deaf community, all he has to do is not wear his processor. What we hope is that he will choose to belong to both worlds, the deaf and the hearing.

For Tania's parents making the decision to allow their daughter to have a cochlear implant, after losing her hearing through meningitis, was an attempt to restore a sensation of hearing of some kind:

> Watching our young daughter suffer this dreadful debilitating illness, leaving the hospital unable to walk, sit up, hold a cup and most devastating unable to hear, and eventually after a few weeks unable to talk, made us determined to do anything and everything within our power to help make some kind of amends to her. When we first heard of cochlear implants at an open information evening we were determined that putting our daughter

back into hospital for a major operation was not the answer for us. At first we were told that she was only partially deaf and that with the help of good hearing aids and lots of patience she would learn to talk. However, it soon became clear not only to us, but also to local professionals that this was not to be the case. It was then decided to try sign language. This too was hard work and although we slowly made some progress we still wanted to hear our little girl talk again. Once more we considered a cochlear implant, only to be told, wrongly, that we must raise the money. Amazingly through the support of our family, friends and the local community we raised enough and took the major step to find out if our daughter was suitable. After the first assessments, we were still not totally convinced that we were 'doing the right thing' so we made contact with an adult who had an implant and it was talking to her that finally made up our minds that this was the right way forward for our daughter.

For Colin's parents the trauma of going back to hospital after the trauma of meningitis, for the medical assessments, before implantation, proved too thought-provoking and they decided that they could not go ahead with the operation. Twelve months later they felt better pre-pared, emotionally, and decided to go ahead with the operation for their young son.

Parents need to be sure in themselves that they are ready to cope with the operation and the ensuing period of tuning and rehabilitation.

For some of the families with older children, what to say to the child can be a major difficulty. Obviously the child is well aware that some-thing is happening. Why all the visits to hospital? How much should parents say and what should they say? The last thing parents want to do is to frighten the child in any way, or to raise hopes too high, just in case anything goes wrong or there are any problems.

Christine's parents agonised for several weeks over how to tell their 9-year-old daughter that all the tests she had undergone at the hospital were leading to an operation for a cochlear implant. Eventually it was decided that Dad should be the one to tell her, while Mum and Christine's older sister went out to do the shopping. With the help of our booklet 'Joanna has a Cochlear Implant' Christine's father was able to explain that she was going to be one of the few special children in the country to receive a very special hearing aid. Not like the ones she was wearing now, but ones that would help her to hear people talking, but she would need to have an operation and she would have to have some of her hair cut off. Dad waited with trepidation for what his daughter was going to say. He wasn't the least bit prepared. 'OK,' she said. When her Mum and sister arrived home she greeted them with

'I'm going to have an operation to have a new hearing aid. Did you know?'
'Yes,' said Mum, who was rather taken aback that her daughter was so mat-ter-of-fact.
'Right,' said Christine, 'I'm going to watch [television] Neighbours now' and ended the conversation.

Kirsty's mother recalls telling her daughter about the imminent operation only to find that the operation posed no apparent problems for her 8-year-old daughter, probably because Mum herself had undergone mastoid surgery at some point and had a scar in the same place as that of an implant operation. Kirsty was only too happy to think that having an operation would help her to hear and talk. However, she was adamant that no one was going to cut off any of her long hair. All the way down to the operating room Kirsty screamed not because of the operation, but because she did not want to lose any of her hair. Loss of hair can be extremely traumatic, especially for the older children and their parents, and this issue needs to be discussed and addressed very carefully by all concerned. All parents are fully aware that the priority must be to reduce the risk of infection, but at the same time, the situation can be dealt with sensitively.

For Anthony's parents the route to obtaining a cochlear implant for their son was even more complex. Anthony was born deaf, and at the time when his parents were contemplating an implant there were no teams in England who would consider implanting a congenitally deaf child. Anthony's family spent lots of time and effort looking at every possibility available for their young son. They started the John Tracy correspondence course and every day Mum sat opposite Anthony doing set activities and giving him all the language to go with them. She sat her son in his rocker on the draining board and talked about dirty cups, the soap bubbles and the clean plates. In her own words 'A fly on the wall would have thought I was completely mad!'

Although he enjoyed these experiences, his parents still felt that it just did not seem to be enough. The family then decided to go to signing class to help give their son a language for communication purposes. A peripatetic teacher visited Anthony at home, but was not in favour of signing and the parents began to realise what a contentious issue this was: to sign or not to sign. An auditory/verbal therapist also began working with Anthony. It was at this point that Anthony's parents first contacted the Nottingham team only to discover that (at that stage) they were only implanting children with acquired deafness. However, Anthony's mother was given the addresses of the New York, Iowa, Hannover and Melbourne programmes and wrote to them all. After numerous tests at a London hospital to find out if Anthony was suitable for an implant at all, Anthony's mother contacted Nottingham again to find out if their policy had changed and enquired whether they would be willing to carry out the rehabilitation, if Anthony had an implant abroad. His mother writes:

In June 1990, we had a reply that they were not yet in a position to implant a congenitally deaf child and neither could they fragment their programme. It is one of the very few occasions that a letter has reduced me to tears.

Eventually, however, it made Anthony's parents even more determined to achieve what they felt was necessary for their son. A visit to the Manhattan Eye, Ear and Throat Hospital and a day spent with the family of an implanted child made the family feel more optimistic, but the prospect of moving to the USA for several years seemed rather daunting. The next to try was the programme in Hannover, which at the time had the most experience of implanting young children. After more tests Anthony was offered an operation in Hannover and the family decided to take up this option. The final decision to implant their congenitally deaf son was not made easily, his mother writes:

> The issue of a congenitally deaf child being born to the deaf community is a huge one which had weighed heavily on my mind for months. I know that Anthony will always be a deaf person and I accept that. I am not trying to change him into a 'hearing' person, but he was born into a hearing family and a hearing world. If he can comprehend even the smallest amount of sound surely it will make life easier for him as an adult in the world at large. He is our child and, like all parents, we can only do what we feel is best for him.

This was perhaps one of the most traumatic routes for any family to have to contemplate to enable their son to have a cochlear implant. It reflects the difficulties encountered by professionals in the UK in starting to introduce programmes for children amidst considerable opposition from parents, professionals and the deaf community. Anthony's parents were fully aware of these problems.

Surgery period

Once the assessments and testing are completed and the decision to go ahead has finally been made, the next hurdle for the family to overcome is the operation itself. In Nottingham the families are encouraged to share the time in hospital together, and on many occasions younger members of the family have accompanied parents in hospital. In the case of one family, mother, new baby and the son who was to be implanted stayed at the hospital, while father, an older daughter and grandparents stayed in a hotel local to the hospital and the family all took it in turns to stay with the patient and to look after the other children. As a family, they felt that the occasion should be shared by all and that no one should feel left out in any way.

At the time of operation, naturally parents are extremely concerned and worried that everything should go well for their child. It is often while their child is in theatre that parents, particularly of children with acquired deafness, re-live their previous hospital experiences. Many parents complained bitterly that they were not well informed about their child's illness, particularly in the case of meningitis and many had left the hospital with no knowledge that their child's hearing was impaired in any way. Several parents recalled instances when they felt they knew their child could no longer hear, before leaving the hospital, but they were not believed or helped by the hospital staff. Many families waited months after their child's illness before the child's hearing was tested and even then they were told that the hearing loss might be temporary or only a partial loss. One mother recalls being told she was 'neurotic' on many occasions because she would not accept the information that her child could hear. After 2 years of numerous appointments her son was declared profoundly deaf. As professionals we need to take note of information given by parents, for they often know their child best.

Perhaps, surprisingly, parents have written very little about the actual time of operation except to make passing comments like James' mother:

> The operation itself is something you worry about from the beginning right up until the time they come out of theatre. Then suddenly it's gone and you get on with the job of helping them to get better, although they seem to do this remarkably quickly with very little help from Mum and Dad. Looking back I think that waiting for the results of the CT scan was just as traumatic as the operation. After all it might have been at this point when it was decided that it just was not possible to go ahead at all.

The children do recover from their operation amazingly quickly; usually after only 48 hours they are up and about, playing in the hospital ward or missing altogether in the case of Kirsty. When visiting the ward only 36 hours after her operation the author found an empty bed and Mum sitting by herself. On enquiring about Kirsty's whereabouts she was told, 'Oh. She's in the stock cupboard helping the nurses to do the stocktaking'. She had made a quick recovery and was back to work!

Initial tuning session

No sooner than the families have overcome the operation and attempted to settle back into the routine of family life, it is time to return to the implant centre for the initial tuning sessions; in the author's programme this involves 3 days in the centre, and makes the initial tuning sessions much less fraught. By the time the family arrive at the centre a visit has already been made to the child's home for them to try on a dummy processor and parents have been reassured that the magnet is working properly. This can be a source of great concern to parents.

On the first day of tuning everyone concerned is anxious, but perhaps the parents most of all. It is at this moment in time when many of them begin to question their decision to have an implant for their child and questions such as 'What if he doesn't like it? What if he won't wear it? What if it doesn't work?' fill their minds. In Barbara's case there was no question about it; she definitely didn't like it and definitely was not going to wear it. Her mother writes:

> On 24 September with great anticipation we went to CHAC for Barbara to be 'switched-on'. We had spent some time trying to tell Barbara what was going to happen and our excitement rubbed off on her. Dressed in her new outfit she had chosen specially for the occasion and full of smiles for everyone, she was 'switched on'. The first sensation of sound distressed Barbara and floods of tears were produced. We came home feeling very flat and disappointed. There was no easy way to overcome this difficulty of Barbara not wanting her head set and processor. At home I sat and nursed Barbara for 20 minutes whilst she sobbed and begged me to take it off. Finally it worked; the next day she cooperated so well at CHAC that we were all delighted

In fact a video was made of this later session and Barbara signs to her mother that she can hear the sounds that the man is making on the computer, and she likes it.

Henry's mother's experience with her son was again somewhat difficult. She writes:

> In the first five minutes Henry showed no response to the testing, although he did seem a little bemused. I'd been prepared for him to hate it and cry but not that it might not work at all! However, after 5 minutes he appeared uncomfortable his eyes started to fill but some excellent tricks by the senior audiologist, introducing a variety of listening games (each one getting more fun and more boisterous) seemed to encourage Henry to tolerate it and respond well. By the end of one and a half hours the scientists had tuned in twenty-one electrodes thereby getting a good basic map for the speech processor. They were very pleased with the progress made.
>
> The afternoon was not so successful, Henry was extremely tired. When I had got the device on and the rehabilitation teacher of the deaf had started playing games with Henry laughing and responding beautifully I was most embarrassed to realise I had not turned it on. Once this had been rectified it was a very different story. We battled with Henry for over an hour but did not manage to keep the device on for more than a few seconds before he screamed and kicked and grabbed it off.
>
> I returned to the hotel at 3.15 p.m. and let Henry play and do his own thing. An hour later I tried again, as had been suggested, on my own. With the television on, the processor was set on one, after an initial struggle he sat quietly and kept it on for fifty minutes during which time I had put it up to three. We looked at some books together. I succeeded again for another fifteen minutes just before he collapsed exhausted in to a deep sleep.

The following 2 days of the initial tuning period were less stressful for Henry and his mother, and on the third day he went home wearing his processor happily.

Not all initial tuning sessions are as fraught as those already mentioned. Alice's parents were most concerned as their daughter had been deafened by meningitis 9 years before her implant, and they

wondered whether or not she would accept the new hearing sensations. Alice's parents were both very nervous on the initial tuning day.
Alice was slightly nervous, but also excited. Alice accepted the sounds
from the computer quite happily and both parents were thrilled to
realise that 16 electrodes had been tuned in a very short time. Over
lunch she wore the processor happily and reacted to several loud environmental sounds and also to her father's voice, when he shouted as
she stepped on his toe. In the afternoon session Alice responded to
many different musical instruments, counting beats and copying
rhythms, although she told us quite precisely what she could and could
not hear. In the evening at the hotel where the family were staying, the
hotelier played the organ for Alice, at first beginning very quietly then
building up the sound until she could hear it. A very happy and satisfy-
ing first day for all the family.

Christine's parents also found that they need not have worried quite
so much as they did. Christine's father remarked that:

> On the first day she was quite happy to wear the processor until bath time
> at 7.30 p.m. She also said that the new 'hearing aid' was better than old
> ones and wanted to wear it again after bath time until bed time, another
> thirty minutes. On day two after the tuning she said the new map was too
> loud, but after ten minutes everything was OK again. In the afternoon she
> had a listening session with the rehabilitation teacher of the deaf and
> responded to voice, drums and a variety of instruments, and was very happy
> with her processor. When we arrived home she played the piano, but com-
> plained that there was too much noise, took the coil off and went for a bath
> (TV had been switched on and with several people talking it may have all
> been too much). After her bath Christine wanted to wear the processor
> again, she responded to voice from about fifteen feet, heard the toilet flush-
> ing and was once again happy with the processor. On the third and final day
> of initial tuning Christine wore her processor all day until bath time, by
> which time we were all very tired!

In Nottingham we are extremely fortunate to have superb accommodation, which can be offered offer to all our families, at the Marjorie
Sherman House (Figure 12.1). The house is situated only a few minutes' walk from the Queen's Medical Centre and was funded by gener-
ous donations made to the supporting charity The Ear Foundation.

Children and their families are able to stay at the house for a very
nominal fee whenever they have an appointment at the Cochlear
Implant Centre. We find the house an invaluable asset to the programme as, working with young children, it is important that the child
arrives at the centre refreshed after a good night's sleep to enable him
or her to cooperate well for the tuning and rehabilitation sessions. As
our families travel from all around the country, the house is an ideal
place to stay.

The three initial days of tuning are very stressful and tiring for all

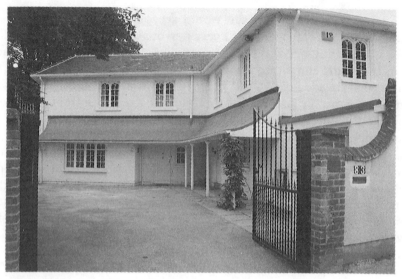

Figure 12.1 Marjorie Sherman house

the family, and it is usually with great relief that they set off for home. Once they are home and get back in to their normal daily routine, the child having accepted the processor and wearing it set at the appropriate sensitivity setting, it then becomes a great temptation to 'test' their child's hearing.

Hayley's father bought a toy drum on his way home from tuning as he had been so impressed by his daughter's obvious pleasure at hearing a drum. However, after several days of banging the drum each time his daughter's attention was elsewhere, she stopped responding! Panic stricken in case there was a problem with the processor he showed the drum to his daughter and asked, using sign language, if she could hear it? 'Yes,' she signed, 'noisy Daddy fed up, stop'.

Nigel's mother was well aware of the fact that she was continually asking her son if he had heard different sounds. One Sunday morning while they were in church someone was playing a guitar, out of Nigel's sight. She asked him what he could hear, he turned and signed to her, 'I know what I can hear and I am not telling you!'.

This made her realise just how often she had asked him this question and she vowed that she would wait in future for him to ask what sounds were, or to tell her himself what a new sound was. Later, he told her he thought he had heard a piano, which was not quite right, as it was a guitar, but an excellent guess.

When the children are first tuned, even if they respond to a sound, it can take many months and sometimes years in the case of the very young children before they can identify a sound consistently. Parents need to be very patient, but also continually aware, so that they can help their children build up a listening library of sounds they know, and encourage them to ask about any new sounds they hear.

In this chapter so far we have discussed with parents:

- The trauma of making the decision to allow their child to have a cochlear implant.
- Preparing the child for the operation.
- The operation time.
- The initial 3 days of tuning.
- The return home.

Learning to listen

It is after the family have returned to their everyday routine that the work of rehabilitation begins, by the families themselves, the local professionals and the implant team. As we have already mentioned, progress initially can be very slow, as Matthew's mother reports:

> At the time of writing it is now over a year since Matthew had his operation and we could never have imagined the stress and worries of the past year. All of our problems have been made easier because we have had constant support and contact with a specialist team. We are lucky in that we are so near the doctors and scientists involved with Matthew, so any checks that Matthew has needed have not involved a plane flight. We know now that to have undertaken this abroad would have added more stress to our lives and especially to Matthew.
>
> The first six months after the operation for us were very difficult. Try as we could to keep our expectations realistic we were watching and wondering what he could hear, and looking for signs of him learning to talk again. It took Matthew three months before he could respond to his name, and his first attempt at Mummy came three months later. We have no regrets in making the decision to have a cochlear implant for Matthew at this crucial stage in his life. He is now saying two and three word phrases and understanding a lot of specific commands and questions. It is important to stress that it is not a magical cure for deafness. Matthew has come a long way during the past year, but he has a long way to go before he can understand general conversation.

Parents have also noticed that their children make good progress and then in Barbara's mother's words:

> We seem to have hit a quiet patch. Have tried for a few days to get Barbara interested in listening games, she made a half hearted attempt at them, but then suggested that we play something else that did not require her to listen. I have tried to think of new listening games, the only one she was enthusiastic about involved the door bell (which has a very loud ring). I also think the past few days have seen less vocalisations.

Then only four days later:

> 'Barbara sang all morning non-stop', she handed me the *Sunday Times* and casually said 'Paper' (not a word we use a lot and not one I have tried to teach her).

Keeping a good sense of humour is very important during the early listening days and Carol's father demonstrates this with the following comments:

> Living where we do, beneath the flight path of Concorde, naturally we were excited when, whilst out walking, Carol looked up in response to the very loud noise made by the aeroplane and signed aeroplane to us. The following week at around the same time we waited anxiously for a repeat performance as Concorde thundered over our heads, nothing! No response!, but then it was foggy!

Christine's parents were very excited when after only 3 months their daughter's name could be called from downstairs, while she was upstairs. Christine's mother called her and waited for the customary reply, 'shut up' but nothing happened, so she called again. This time she did get an answer 'I'm on the toilet!', a place where she obviously was not used to being disturbed.

Many parents consider that their deaf child may be safer if they learn to use an implant. Angela's mother feels quite strongly that Angela's ability to hear helped save her life:

> The implant saved Angela's life today. We were crossing the road when a car came out of nowhere, I shouted at Angela to stop as she was ahead of me. If she had not had the implant she would have been dead by now. The car was travelling at about 80–90 mph. She is taking a lot more care on the road now.

Six months later the same mother writes:

> Angela phoned Jean (her taxi escort) to say that she was going to school tomorrow, Angela had been poorly since Tuesday. She dialled Jean's number and said 'I'm going to school tomorrow Jean'. Angela asked Jean what time she would pick her up and Jean said 8 'o'clock'. I asked Angela what time she said and Angela said 8 'o'clock'. Jean was thrilled she said she understood every word that Angela had said, and she went around telling everyone about it.

Learning how to use the telephone can take lots of patience and lots of practice, so we do encourage parents to allow their children to answer the telephone, when it rings, very soon after the initial tuning. However, as Hayley's Mum reports this can sometimes create problems:

> The telephone rang tonight. I told Hayley it was ringing and she ran to answer it. She talked for 3–4 minutes non-stop and then replaced the receiver! Luckily it was a friend who telephoned straight back and was thrilled to hear Hayley trying to talk.

Advice from Barbara's mother is:

> Make sure you inform all your family and friends that you are helping your child to learn to listen for the telephone ringing, because on several

occasions when we have asked Barbara what she could hear, she has correctly said the telephone, but sometimes we have let it ring for so long to see if she will tell us it is ringing, that people have rung off and we are still waiting for a call.

Learning how to use the telephone proficiently can take a long time and requires lots of practice. David, one of our older implantees, did not enjoy his telephone training saying it was 'too difficult'. One morning he asked his mother if his friend could accompany him to a local football match. 'Yes I suppose so,' she said, 'Why don't you ring and ask him?' Without thinking about it David picked up the telephone and rang his friend while his Mum waited anxiously in the kitchen. Five minutes later he appeared at the door saying, 'His Mum says he can't come, because he's still in bed!' David did not realise why his mother was so thrilled that his friend was not going to the match; he had understood what had been said over the telephone in a situation meaningful to him rather than a 'test' one.

Special moments

As any child grows up there are many special moments which parents record not only on paper, but also in their hearts. Parents who have children with cochlear implants are no different but the special moments they recall may be slightly different.

Jamie's Mum says:

He is responding to many sounds, he turns to his name, he loves music, he's heard wind whistling in the trees, he's heard birds singing, he's constantly asking us what different sounds are, and his speech is improving all the time.

While David's mother reports:

He can identify most household sounds, respond to his name immediately and can follow some of a conversation without lipreading. He is just learning to listen to music and his favourite is Tina Turner at its loudest volume! He is able to be part of a mainstream class and copes well with the demands of school.

For Matthew's mother these words were very special:

Last week as I was leaving Matthew's bedroom he said 'Door, no leave it' which may not seem unusual but they are words we thought we would never hear again along with 'Night, night Mummy, I love you'.

For Tania's parents it wasn't even a sentence:

The girls were washed and dressed this morning and had just cleaned their teeth as always. I said to Billie open your mouth (so I could inspect the teeth) and say 'aah'. On Tania's turn she obliged with the open mouth and out came a very high pitched 'aah', we were overwhelmed. It was only a matter of months ago we took her to the doctor's, he had asked her to say 'aah' and we had said to him if only she could!

Carol's mother witnessed an impromptu concert in her back garden one morning, when she asked her daughter what she was doing waving her arms around; she signed that she was listening to the birds singing and she was conducting the performance.

Barbara's mother writes:

> Tear jerker of the week coming up. Last week was my birthday and Barbara sang 'Happy Birthday' with no prompting. Although the words were not yet recognisable the tune certainly was.

The special moments are endless as with all growing children. In the Nottingham programme we find it extremely useful to ask the parents of our implanted children to recall, at the 1-year, 2-year and 3-year postimplant stages, what they feel would be the most important considerations for other prospective parents of implanted children, before making the decision to go ahead with implantation for their child. Overwhelmingly many parents felt that obtaining as much information from as many different people as possible was by far the most important consideration. Having realistic expectations and realising the time it takes for progress to show, particularly with the young children, was also stressed by many parents. Perhaps most important was the need to feel that the parents had made up their own minds in the light of information given.

By far the most common responses by parents of implanted children were the following:

- Get as much information as possible and speak to other parents.
- If there is anything that you are unsure of, ask.
- Be prepared for slow progress, don't expect miracles.
- Try to satisfy every little doubt and worry that you have; no question is too trivial.
- Parents *must* give the input following implantation and get information on how to do it.
- Try to attend an implant information day.
- Make up your own mind.

Perhaps the final word should come from a child with a cochlear implant. When asked his opinion about what advice he would give to a parent contemplating cochlear implantation for their child his comment was:

> Don't waste any time, get the operation done and let the fun begin!

This same child was asked by his mainstream class teacher to write about a change which had occurred in his life. After thinking carefully he chose to write about how having a cochlear implant had changed his life. His unedited version is shown in Figure 12.2.

Parents on the author's programme are scattered far and wide around the country and, although a telephone call to the parent of another implanted child can help tremendously to ease a worried mind, meeting with other families is a great support for children and parents alike. Talking to parents who have shared a similar experience can be extremely helpful. Formal and informal gatherings (Figure 12.3) are organised at frequent intervals throughout the years; some include

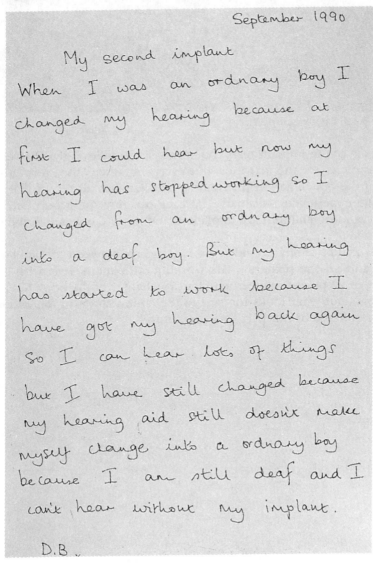

September 1990

My second implant

When I was an ordnary boy I changed my hearing because at first I could hear but now my hearing has stopped working so I changed from an ordnary boy into a deaf boy. But my hearing has started to work because I have got my hearing back again so I can hear lots of things but I have still changed because my hearing aid still doesn't make myself change into a ordnary boy because I am still deaf and I can't hear without my implant.

D.B.

Figure 12.2 A child's story

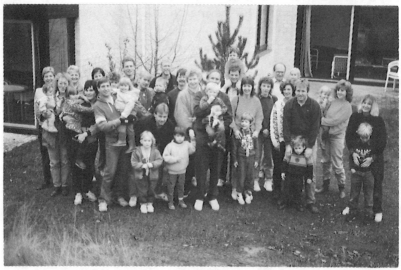

Figure 12.3 Family group

members of the implant team, others are for families only. The venues
are varied as are the activities, but everyone agrees they form a vital
part of the rehabilitation programme, and families all report that they
find the experiences invaluable. At each meeting the group becomes
larger as more children are implanted and more families join the programme.

The child's family provides the crucial link between the implanted
child and all the professionals working with them. It is with great
thanks to all parents concerned that this chapter of the book has been
possible. Out team looks forward to the continuation of the excellent
support offered by our parents in the future.

Index